Intellectual and Developmental Disabilities Nursing

Scope and Standards of Practice

3rd Edition

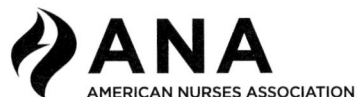

The American Nurses Association (ANA) is a national professional association. This publication reflects the position of ANA regarding the scope and standards of intellectual and developmental disability nursing practice and should be reviewed in conjunction with state board of nursing regulations. State law, rules, and regulations govern the practice of nursing, while *Intellectual and Developmental Disability Nursing: Scope and Standards of Practice, 3rd Edition* guides registered nurses in the application of their professional skills and responsibilities.

About the American Nurses Association
The American Nurses Association (ANA) is the only full-service professional organization representing the interests of the nation's 4.2 million registered nurses through its constituent/state nurses associations and its organizational affiliates. The ANA advances the nursing profession by fostering high standards of nursing practice, promoting the rights of nurses in the workplace, projecting a positive and realistic view of nursing, and by lobbying the Congress and regulatory agencies on health care issues affecting nurses and the public.

American Nurses Association
8515 Georgia Avenue, Suite 400
Silver Spring, MD 20910

Copyright © 2022 ANA. All rights reserved. No part of this book may be reproduced or used in any form or any means, electronic or mechanical, including photocopying and recording, or by any information storage and retrieval system, without permission in writing from the publisher.

ISBNs
Print 978-1-947800-89-2
ePDF 978-1-947800-90-8
ePUB 978-1-947800-91-5
Mobi 978-1-947800-92-2
SAN: 851-3481

Contents

Contributors • vii
    ANA Committee on Nursing Practice Standards   vii
    ANA Staff   vii
    About This Publication   vii
    About the American Nurses Association   vii

Overview of the Content • xi
    Essential Documents of Professional Nursing   xi
    Additional Content   xii
    Audience for This Publication   xiii

IDD Nursing Scope of Practice • 1
    Definition of Nursing   1
    Definition of Intellectual and Developmental Disability (IDD) Nursing   2
        Description of the Scope of IDD Nursing Practice   3
    Specialty Practice in IDD Nursing   5
    Development and Function of IDD Nursing Standards of
       Professional Practice   8
        Standards of Professional Nursing Practice in IDD   8
        Standards of Practice in IDD Nursing   8
        Standards of Professional Performance in IDD Nursing   9
        The Function of Competencies in IDD Nursing Standards   11
    What Is IDD Nursing?   11
    When Nursing Occurs   15
    The How of IDD Nursing   16
    Integrating the Science and Art of IDD Nursing   17
    The Art of IDD Nursing   18
        Care and Caring in IDD Nursing Practice   19
        Cultural Components of Care   21
    The Science of IDD Nursing   22
        IDD Nursing Knowledge   22

    Research in IDD Nursing   26
    Evidence-Based Practice in IDD Nursing   28
  The Where of IDD Nursing Practice   29
    Healthy Work Environments for Nursing Practice   31
      Safe Patient Handling and Mobility (SPHM)   32
      Fatigue in Nursing Practice   34
      Workplace Violence and Incivility   35
      Optimal Staffing   36
    Supports for Healthy Work Environments   37
      American Nurses Association   37
      American Association of Critical Care Nurses Standards   38
  High-Performing Interprofessional Teams   39
  Key Influences on the Quality and Environment of Nursing Practice   40
  Societal, Cultural, and Ethical Dimensions Describe the Why and How of IDD Nursing   41
  The Code of Ethics for Nurses   43
  Professional Registered Nurses Today: The Who of IDD Nursing   50
    Statistical Snapshot   50
      Licensure and Education of IDD Registered Nurses   51
  Definitions and Concepts Related to Competence in IDD Nursing   53
    Evaluating Competence   55

Professional Trends and Issues • 57
  Creating a Sustainable Nursing Workforce   59
  Nursing Education   61
  Technological Advances   62
  Population Focus   65
    Redefining Health and Well-Being for the Millennial Generation   65
    Baby Boomers: Health and Chronic Illness   66
  Summary of the Scope of IDD Nursing Practice   69

Standards of Professional Nursing Practice • 71
  Significance of Standards   71

Standards of Practice for IDD Nurses • 72
  Standard 1. Assessment   72
    Competencies   72

Additional competencies for the graduate-level prepared
  registered nurse who specializes in IDD   74
Additional competencies for the APRN who specializes in IDD   74
Standard 2. Diagnosis   74
  Competencies   74
    Additional competencies for the graduate-level prepared
      registered nurse who specializes in IDD   75
    Additional competencies for the APRN who specializes in IDD   75
Standard 3. Outcomes Identification   76
  Competencies   76
    Additional competencies for the graduate-level prepared
      registered nurse who specializes in IDD, including the APRN
      who specializes in IDD   77
Standard 4. Planning   77
  Competencies   77
    Additional competencies for the graduate-level prepared
      registered nurse who specializes in IDD   79
    Additional competencies for the APRN who specializes in IDD   79
Standard 5. Implementation   80
  Competencies   80
    Additional competencies for the graduate-level prepared
      registered nurse who specializes in IDD   81
    Additional competencies for the APRN who specializes in IDD   82
Standard 5A. Coordination of Care   83
  Competencies   83
    Additional competencies for the graduate-level prepared
      registered nurse who specializes in IDD   84
    Additional competencies for the APRN who specializes in IDD   84
Standard 5B. Health Teaching and Health Promotion   85
  Competencies   85
    Additional competencies for the graduate-level prepared
      registered nurse, including the APRN who specializes in IDD   86
Standard 6. Evaluation   86
  Competencies   86
    Additional competencies for the graduate-level prepared
      registered nurse, including the APRN who specializes in IDD   87

Standards of Professional Performance for IDD Nurses • 88
    Standard 7. Ethics   88
        Competencies   88
            Additional competencies for the APRN who specializes in IDD   91
    Standard 8. Culturally Congruent Practice   92
        Competencies   92
            Additional competencies for the graduate-level prepared registered nurse   93
            Additional competencies for the APRN   93
    Standard 9. Communication   94
        Competencies   94
    Standard 10. Collaboration   95
        Competencies   95
            Additional competencies for the APRN who specializes in IDD   96
    Standard 11. Leadership   97
        Competencies   97
            Additional competencies for the APRN who specializes in IDD   98
    Standard 12. Education   99
        Competencies   99
    Standard 13. Evidence-Based Practice and Research   100
        Competencies   100
            Additional competencies for the APRN who specializes in IDD   101
    Standard 14. Quality of Practice   102
        Competencies   102
            Additional competencies for the APRN who specializes in IDD   103
    Standard 15. Professional Practice Evaluation   103
        Competencies   103
            Additional competencies for the APRN who specializes in IDD   104
    Standard 16. Resource Utilization   104
        Competencies   104
            Additional competencies for the APRN who specializes in IDD   106
    Standard 17. Environmental Health   106
        Competencies   106
            Additional competencies for the APRN who specializes in IDD   107

Glossary • 109
References • 121
Index • 135

Contributors

The American Nurses Association (ANA) thanks those who contributed their valuable time and talents to development of *Intellectual and Developmental Disabilities Nursing: Scope and Standards of Practice,* 3rd Edition. This resource builds on and replaces previous editions entitled *Intellectual and Developmental Disabilities Nursing: Scope and Standards of Practice* and the original *Statement on the Scope and Standards for the Nurse Who Specializes in Developmental Disabilities and/or Mental Retardation.* The terminology has changed over the years and is reflected in each edition of the scope statement and standards of this specialty nursing practice.

The authors of *Intellectual and Developmental Disabilities Nursing: Scope and Standards of Practice,* 3rd Edition, involved persons with disabilities and family members of individuals with disabilities and include:

Cecily L. Betz, PhD, RN, FAAN, Chair, University of Southern California, University Center for Excellence in Developmental Disabilities, Children's Hospital Los Angeles; Task Force Member, IDD Nursing: Scope and Standards, 1st, 2nd Edition

Jennifer Adams, EdM, MSN, RN, ACCNS-P, CPN, CNE, Society of Pediatric Nurses (SPN) Representative

Karen W. Burkett, PhD, RN, PPCNP-BC, Division of Developmental and Behavioral Pediatrics; Leadership Education in Neurodevelopmental Disabilities (LEND), Cincinnati Children's Hospital Medical Center

Wendy A. Chouteau, DNP, APRN, FNP-BC, Division of Neurology/Comprehensive Neuromuscular Center, Cincinnati Children's Hospital Medical Center

Louvisia "Lou" A. Conley MEd, EdS, Boling Center for Developmental Disabilities

Eduardo del Rosario, PhD Student, FNP-BC, Barbara H. Hagan School of Nursing and Health Sciences, Molloy College

Jean Farley, DNP, RN, PNP-BC, Georgetown University, School of Nursing and Health Studies

Veronica Feeg, PhD, RN, FAAN, Barbara H. Hagan School of Nursing and Health Sciences, Molloy College

Laurie Fleming, MPH, RN, NCSN, National Association of School Nurses (NASN) Representative

Michelle S. Franklin, PhD, MSN, FNP-BC, PMHNP-BC, CNS, Carolina Institute for Developmental Disabilities, University of North Carolina at Chapel Hill

J. Carolyn Graff, PhD, RN, FAAIDD, University of Tennessee Health Science Center, Boling Center for Developmental Disabilities

Marilyn Krajicek, EdD, RN, FAAN, University of Colorado College of Nursing; Task Force Member, IDD Nursing: Scope and Standards, 1st, 2nd Edition

Rebecca Kronk, PhD, MSN, CRNP, FAAN, CNE, ANEF, International Society of Nurses in Genetics (ISONG) Representative

Lindsey Minchella, MSN, RN, NCSN, FNASN, National Association of School Nurses (NASN) Representative

S. Diane Moore, BSN, RN, CDDN, Developmental Disabilities Nurses Association (DDNA) Representative

Wendy M. Nehring, PhD, RN, FAAN, FAAIDD, Chair, Task Force IDD Nursing: Scope and Standards, 1st, 2nd Edition; East Tennessee State University, College of Nursing

Teresa A. Savage, PhD, RN, Department of Women, Children & Family Health Science, College of Nursing, University of Illinois at Chicago; Task Force Member, IDD Nursing: Scope and Standards, 1st, 2nd Edition

Nhu Tran, RN, PhD, MSN, CCRN, CCRP, Academy of Neonatal Nurses Representative

Susan Van Cleve, DNP, RN, CPNP-PC, PMHS, FAANP, FAAN, National Association of Pediatric Nurse Practitioners (NAPNAP) Representative

Cassandra Wolf, BSN, RN, Cincinnati Children's Hospital Medical Center

ANA COMMITTEE ON NURSING PRACTICE STANDARDS

Mona Pearl Treyball, PhD, RN, CNS, CCRN-K, FAAN (Co-Chair February 2019–December 2020)
Stacy McNall, MSN, RN, IBCLC, PMHNP-BC (Co-Chair February 2020–December 2021)
Patricia Bowe, DNP, MS, RN
Nena M. Bonuel, PhD, RN, APRN-BC, ACNS-BC, CCRN-K
Danette Culver, MSN, RN, APRN, ACNS-BC, CCRN-K
Elizabeth "Liz" O. Dietz, EdD, RN, CS-NP, CSN
Tonette "Toni" McAndrew, MPA, RN
Amy McCarthy, MSN, RN, RNC-MNN, NE-BC
Linda Inez Perkins, MSN, RN-BC (Alternate)
Shelly Wells, PhD, MBA, APRN-CNS, ANEF (Alternate)

ANA STAFF

Carol Bickford, PhD, RN-BC, CPHIMS, FAMIA, FHIMSS, FAAN (content editor)
Erin Walpole, BA, PMP (project editor)

ABOUT THIS PUBLICATION

In September 2020, ANA's Board of Directors approved the scope statement and acknowledged the standards of practice and professional performance of *Intellectual and Developmental Disabilities Nursing: Scope and Standards of Practice*, 3rd Edition, as defined herein. Approval is valid for five years from the first date of publication of this document or until a new scope of practice has been approved, whichever occurs first.

ABOUT THE AMERICAN NURSES ASSOCIATION

The American Nurses Association (ANA) is the only full-service professional organization representing the interests of the nation's 4.2 million registered nurses through its constituent or state nurses associations and its organizational affiliates. ANA advances the nursing profession by fostering high standards of nursing practice, promoting the rights of nurses in the workplace, projecting a positive and realistic view of nursing, and lobbying the Congress and regulatory agencies on healthcare issues affecting nurses and the public.

Overview of the Content

ESSENTIAL DOCUMENTS OF PROFESSIONAL NURSING

ANA has been the vanguard for nursing practice for more than a century. The *Code of Ethics for Nurses with Interpretive Statements* (ANA, 2015b) and *Nursing: Scope and Standards of Practice* (3rd ed.; ANA, 2015a) are documents produced by ANA to inform the thinking and decision-making of registered nurses practicing in the United States and guide their practice. The *Code of Ethics for Nurses with Interpretive Statements* (ANA, 2015b) lists the nine succinct provisions that establish the ethical framework for registered nurses across all roles, levels, and settings. *Nursing: Scope and Standards of Practice* (3rd ed.; ANA, 2015a) outlines the expectations of the professional role of the registered nurse. It includes the Scope of Nursing Practice Statement and presents the Standards of Professional Nursing Practice and their accompanying competencies. These documents are intended to help provide the public with assurances of safe and competent nursing care.

Along with these documents, specialty nursing organizations have worked with ANA to publish specific standards of professional practice in their specialty. This document, concerning the care of individuals with intellectual and developmental disabilities (hereafter referred to as IDD), is a revision of the *Intellectual and Developmental Nursing: Scope and Standards of Practice*, 2nd Edition. This document has been revised to:

- capture the changing practice of nursing in this specialty (i.e., encompassing all levels of education and all system levels of care from the individual to the system itself),

- emphasize the unique healthcare needs and characteristics of individuals of all ages with IDD,
- incorporate the ANA standards mentioned earlier (ANA, 2015a),
- incorporate the provisions of the *Code of Ethics for Nurses with Interpretive Statements* (ANA, 2015b),
- emphasize the importance of a family-centered and consumer-centered framework of care, and
- incorporate the developments in the field since the last edition.

The previous edition of these specialty standards and scope of practice is found on ANA's website, Nursingworld.org.

Adolescents and adults with IDD and their families or legal guardians engage in shared decision-making with healthcare professionals to make person-centered decisions about their health care. This self-advocacy has arisen in tandem with an evolving healthcare system that may or may not optimize healthcare options for all people. Therefore, in response to these changes, individuals of all ages and abilities with IDD and their families or legal guardians should be assured of safe and effective nursing care. This document addresses this care, the associated nursing standards, and the competencies expected of registered nurses who specialize in IDD practices.

ADDITIONAL CONTENT

This document should also be used in conjunction with other specialty nursing scope and standards of practice and professional performance such as but not limited to *Pediatric Nursing: Scope and Standards of Practice*, 2nd Edition (Society of Pediatric Nurses [SPN], National Association of Pediatric Nurse Practitioners [NAPNAP], & ANA, 2015); *Genetics-Genomics Nursing: Scope and Standards of Practice*, 2nd Edition (International Society of Nurses in Genetics, Inc. [ISONG] & ANA, 2016); *Public Health Nursing: Scope and Standards of Practice*, 2nd Edition (ANA, 2013a); *Psychiatric-Mental Health Nursing: Scope and Standards of Practice*, 2nd Edition (American Psychiatric Nurses Association, International Society of Psychiatric-Mental Health Nurses, & ANA, 2014); and *School

Nursing: Scope and Standards of Practice, 3rd Edition (National Association of School Nurses [NASN] & ANA, 2017). Additional important nursing documents that address the history and context of nursing standards include *Nursing: Scope and Standards of Practice*, 3rd Edition (ANA, 2015a); *Principles of Environmental Health for Nursing Practice* (ANA, 2007a); *Professional Role Competence: ANA Position Statement* (ANA, 2014b); and *Principles for Nursing Documentation for Registered Nurses and Professional Nursing* (ANA, 2010b).

AUDIENCE FOR THIS PUBLICATION

Nurses of any educational level and employed in any setting that serves individuals of any age with IDD make up the primary audience for this book. Legislators, regulators, legal counsel, and the judiciary system will also want to reference it. Agencies, organizations, nurse administrators, other nurses not working in this specialty, and other interprofessional colleagues will find this publication an invaluable reference. In addition, healthcare consumers with IDD, their families or legal guardians, communities, and populations using healthcare and nursing services that cover the care of persons with IDD can use this document to better understand the role and responsibilities of registered nurses and advanced practice registered nurses (APRNs) who specialize in IDD.

IDD Nursing Scope of Practice

Many nurses are unfamiliar with this unique specialty nursing practice area because the intellectual and developmental disability (IDD) nursing specialty historically was primarily associated with an institutional setting and the stigma attached to this population until the late 1950s. In fact, this nursing specialty was only recognized by ANA in 1997 (Nehring, 1999). Unlike many nursing specialties, the scope of practice for nurses who specialize in IDD extends across all levels of care and all healthcare and many educational settings. Even though healthcare consumers with IDD are present today in all communities and healthcare settings, they remain a vulnerable and marginalized population. Many healthcare professionals are not educated or prepared to care for specific condition-related and developmental needs of individuals with IDD. Such health disparities were highlighted in the Surgeon General's report, *Closing the Gap: A National Blueprint for Improving the Health of Persons with Mental Retardation* (U.S. Public Health Service, 2002). Working in an interdisciplinary context, nurses continue to strive to promote the importance of the nursing contribution in this specialty field and to provide health care at both the generalist and advanced practice level.

DEFINITION OF NURSING

Nursing is the protection, promotion, and optimization of health and abilities, prevention of illness and injury, facilitation of healing, alleviation of suffering through the diagnosis and treatment of human response, and advocacy in the care of individuals, families, groups, communities, and populations. (ANA, 2015a, p. 1)

This definition serves as the foundation for the following expanded description of the Scope of Nursing Practice and the Standards of Professional Nursing Practice for nurses who specialize in IDD.

DEFINITION OF INTELLECTUAL AND DEVELOPMENTAL DISABILITY (IDD) NURSING

Consistent with the ANA (2015a) definition of nursing, IDD nursing focuses on protecting, promoting, and optimizing the health and functioning ability of persons with IDD; diagnosing and treating persons with IDD to maximize their quality of life and alleviate discomfort and suffering; and advocating for and with persons with IDD and their families within and across groups, communities, and society.

Nurses who practice in the specialty field of IDD have clinical expertise and experience pertaining to the illness–health continuum of care of individuals across the life course whose conditions meet the diagnostic criteria identified in the Developmental Disabilities Assistance and Bill of Rights Act of 2000 (Box 1). IDD nursing practice is based upon a family-centered and, in later years, an individual-centered philosophy of care wherein the family (and when appropriate, the individual) are considered full partners in the development of the comprehensive plan of care. IDD nursing is comprehensive in scope and is focused on all aspects of the biopsychosocial needs of the person with IDD, their family, and their community, as well as the resources that are available to the person, family, and community.

Major biopsychosocial issues impacting individuals with IDD and of ongoing concern for IDD nurses and their interprofessional colleagues include:

- Primary, secondary, and tertiary prevention of developmental disability (DD) and intellectual disability (ID);
- Community inclusion;
- Transition from pediatric to adult DD services;
- Expansion of services that promote independence beyond their 22nd birthday;
- Access to high-quality, community-based health care, including a health home;

- Provision of culturally relevant care across the spectrum of IDD nursing;
- Health equity;
- Social determinants of health; and
- Nondiscrimination in educational and work settings.

Description of the Scope of IDD Nursing Practice

Nurse members of the American Association on Intellectual and Developmental Disabilities (AAIDD), Developmental Disabilities Nurses Association (DDNA), American Academy of Developmental Medicine and Dentistry (AADMD), and other professional nursing associations have deemed it important that there be a scope and standards of practice for this specialty. This document serves as the contemporary template for the practice of nursing in IDD, and the standards of practice portion of this document serves as a description of the practice of nurses who specialize in this field.

IDD nurses help comprehensively manage the biopsychosocial needs of children and adults with IDD in a wide array of health and community settings. IDD nursing is practiced in settings that may not be consistently germane to other nursing specialties, such as early intervention programs; special education programs in preschool, elementary, middle, and high schools; postsecondary college and vocational programs; group homes; mental health programs; correctional facilities; and long-term care, senior residential, and support programs. IDD nurses serve as care consultants for nursing specialties, nurse educators, nurse researchers, and interprofessional colleagues when they work with individuals with IDD. IDD consultation efforts include assistance with the provision of the care that addresses the unique care needs for patients with IDD who are hospitalized in tertiary and subacute settings. IDD nurses can be consulted about the provision of referrals to available resources and community services for those with IDD. IDD nurses can coordinate care and establish wraparound support networks from a wide array of resources, including clinics, hospitals, rehabilitation facilities, schools, transportation, supported employment, mental and behavioral programs, and housing. The

BOX 1. DEFINITION OF DEVELOPMENTAL DISABILITY

DEVELOPMENTAL DISABILITIES ASSISTANCE AND BILL OF RIGHTS ACT OF 2000

(A) IN GENERAL. The term "developmental disability" means a severe, chronic disability of an individual that
- (i) is attributable to a mental or physical impairment or combination of mental and physical impairments;
- (ii) is manifested before the individual attains age 22;
- (iii) is likely to continue indefinitely;
- (iv) results in substantial functional limitations in three or more of the following areas of major life activity:
  - (I) Self-care.
  - (II) Receptive and expressive language.
  - (III) Learning.
  - (IV) Mobility.
  - (V) Self-direction.
  - (VI) Capacity for independent living.
  - (VII) Economic self-sufficiency.
- (v) reflects the individual's need for a combination and sequence of special, interdisciplinary, or generic services, individualized supports, or other forms of assistance that are of lifelong or extended duration and are individually planned and coordinated.

(B) INFANTS AND YOUNG CHILDREN. An individual from birth to age nine, inclusive, who has a substantial developmental delay or specific congenital or acquired condition, may be considered to have a developmental disability without meeting three or more of the criteria described in clauses (i) through (v) of subparagraph (A) if the individual, without services and supports, has a high probability of meeting those criteria later in life.

uniqueness of IDD nursing is that IDD nurses complete care coordination that is complex involving resources from a myriad of agencies and organizations that are not characteristically accessed in clinical settings. Furthermore, IDD nurses recognize resources that are available through local, state, regional, and national governing bodies.

The scope of IDD nursing practice is consistent with the 2015 ANA Scope and Standards of Practice (2015a), which describes the "who," "what," "where," "when," "why," and "how" of nursing practice. The answer to each of these questions helps to provide a complete picture of the dynamic and complex practice of IDD nursing. The definition of nursing answers the "what" of the nursing practice question. IDD nurses are registered nurses and APRNs "who" have been educated, credentialed, and maintain active licensure to practice nursing. IDD nursing occurs "when" there is a need for nursing knowledge, wisdom, caring, leadership, practice, or education that is specific to persons with IDD and their families and those who care for them. IDD nursing occurs in any environment or setting "where" there is a person with IDD in need of care, information, or advocacy. The "how" of IDD nursing practice refers to the ways, means, methods, and manners that IDD nurses use to practice professionally. The "why" is characterized as IDD nursing's response to the changing needs of society to achieve positive healthcare outcomes for persons with IDD aligned with nursing's social contract with an obligation to society. The full spectrum of the IDD nurse's role in this specialty is described for both the registered nurse and APRN. The depth and breadth with which individual registered nurses and APRNs engage in the total scope of IDD nursing practice for this specialty depend on each nurse's education, experience, role, and the population served.

SPECIALTY PRACTICE IN IDD NURSING

All nurses will care for an individual with IDD sometime in their career. Each person with IDD is a person first, and each person's healthcare needs are unique. It is important that nurses recognize that a person with IDD (a) is not unwell based on the diagnosis of IDD, (b) does not necessarily have all of the secondary conditions identified as common to the diagnosis (e.g., a person with spina bifida does not always have hydrocephaly), and (c) experiences many of the same life events (e.g., graduation, first job, etc.) and has the same feelings that all individuals have. It is important that diagnostic overshadowing does not occur. Diagnostic overshadowing refers to attributing a health problem to the person's diagnosis of IDD. For example, an adolescent with hydrocephalus who arrives in the emergency room with headbanging behavior does not automatically have a shunt malfunction; they could be in pain or have constipation (Reiss, Levitan, & Szyszko, 1982).

Registered nurses must be able to provide care to individuals with IDD, but in most nursing education programs, the curricular content and clinical experiences related to the care of persons with IDD are minimal. All levels of nursing education should include content about IDD and clinical experiences should include individuals with IDD. Nurses practicing as registered nurses, both at the undergraduate and graduate level, must be able to provide holistic care to this population. Many books, articles, videos, and internet sites are available to assist in this learning. Additionally, professional organizations such as DDNA, AAIDD, AADMD, and the National Association of School Nurses (NASN) support continued development of the nurse caring for those with IDD.

School nurses follow the definition of school nursing (NASN, 2017a,b) for all students, including students with IDD, to protect and promote their health, facilitate their optimal development, and advance their academic success. School nurses bridge the healthcare and education systems for students with IDD, coordinate their care, advocate for student-centered care, and collaborate to design systems that allow individuals with IDD to develop to their full potential (NASN, 2017a,b).

The registered nurse who specializes in IDD provides care to individuals across the life course. Care of the persons with IDD should include families or legal guardians, particularly if individuals are unable to make their own decisions or actively participate in their own care. School nurses are responsible for clear and consistent communication channels among school personnel, students, parents or guardians, healthcare providers, and teachers. This is an essential role of school nurses that promotes health stability and progress in working with students with IDD and their families.

IDD registered nurses, including APRNs, are included in an interprofessional team for healthcare consumers with IDD and are responsible for the coordination of care and support for individuals with IDD. The IDD registered nurse participates in the implementation of individual and family or legal guardians' assessment and in the planning, implementation, and evaluation of their health and health services with the healthcare consumer with IDD, family or legal guardians, and community support staff as partners. School nurses are members of the Individualized Educational Program (IEP) and Individualized Family Service Plan (IFSP) teams and use the nursing process to provide healthcare guidance to team members including students, parents, teachers, therapists, and administrators to develop the IEP or IFSP, provide services, as directed by that plan, and update the plan regularly (Betz, 2017; Betz, Krajicek, & Craft-Rosenberg, 2018; Institute of Medicine [IOM], 2001; SPN, NAP-NAP, & ANA, 2015).

Additionally, all IDD registered nurses have roles in the preparation of youth as they transition to adult care. Recommendations for such preparations have been published by key organizations, including the American Academy of Pediatrics (AAP), the American Academy of Family Physicians (AAFP), the American College of Physicians (ACP) (AAP, AAFP, ACP-ASIM, 2002; Cooley, Sagerman, et al., 2011; White et al., 2018), the American Society of Internal Medicine (Talente & LeComte, 2013), the Society of Adolescent Medicine (Blum et al., 1993; Rosen, 2003), and position statements published by the Society of Pediatric Nursing (SPN) (Betz, 2017), NAPNAP (2020), and the NASN (2019a). School nurses work with and advocate for children and youth, parents, and their staff as students transition from home to preschool, preschool to primary school, primary to middle school, middle school to high school, and high school to adulthood. For the latter, they help to make transitions smooth by beginning to utilize procedures (e.g., medication administration) that will be similar in adulthood and connect families with agencies and programs that may provide services to the student in adulthood.

DEVELOPMENT AND FUNCTION OF IDD NURSING STANDARDS OF PROFESSIONAL PRACTICE

The Standards of Professional Nursing Practice in IDD Nursing are authoritative statements of the responsibilities that all registered nurses in this specialty are expected to perform competently (ANA, 2015a). These standards serve as evidence of the standard of care for IDD nursing with the understanding that their application depends on context. The standards of professional practice in IDD nursing are subject to change as specific conditions and clinical circumstances change, and new patterns of professional practice are developed and accepted by the nursing profession and the public. These standards will be formally and periodically reviewed and revised.

Standards of Professional Nursing Practice in IDD

The Standards of Professional Nursing Practice in IDD include the Standards of Practice and the Standards of Professional Performance in IDD.

Standards of Practice in IDD Nursing

A competent level of IDD nursing care is demonstrated by the nursing process, which includes assessment, diagnosis, outcomes identification, planning, implementation, and evaluation. Consistent with ANA scope and standards of practice for nurses (2015a), IDD registered nurses engage in the nursing process, which is the foundation of the nurse's decision-making.

STANDARD 1. ASSESSMENT: The IDD registered nurse collects data related to the health and the environmental situation or barriers of the person with IDD.

STANDARD 2. DIAGNOSIS: The IDD registered nurse analyzes the assessment data to determine the actual or potential diagnoses, problems and issues, and strengths and assets of the healthcare consumer with IDD.

STANDARD 3. OUTCOMES IDENTIFICATION: The IDD registered nurse identifies expected outcomes for a plan that is individualized to the healthcare consumer with IDD and the situation.

STANDARD 4. PLANNING: The IDD registered nurse develops a plan that prescribes strategies and alternatives to reach expected measurable outcomes.

STANDARD 5. IMPLEMENTATION: The IDD registered nurse implements the identified plan.

STANDARD 5A. COORDINATION OF CARE: The IDD registered nurse coordinates care delivery that requires the nurse to work closely with individuals with IDD, families, community resources, and health systems.

STANDARD 5B. HEALTH TEACHING AND HEALTH PROMOTION: The IDD registered nurse uses strategies to promote health, prevention of secondary disability, and a safe environment for individuals with IDD.

STANDARD 6. EVALUATION: The IDD registered nurse evaluates progress toward attainment of goals and outcomes of individuals with IDD and their families.

Standards of Professional Performance in IDD Nursing

The Standards of Professional Performance, which describe a competent level of behavior for all registered nurses in their role as a professional nurse, apply equally to all IDD registered nurses in their professional role activities. IDD registered nurses are expected to engage in professional role activities that are appropriate to and consistent with their education and their position. As with all registered nurses, IDD registered nurses are accountable for their professional behavior to themselves, healthcare consumers with IDD families or legal guardians of healthcare consumers with IDD, their professional peers, and society (ANA, 2015a).

STANDARD 7. ETHICS: The IDD registered nurse practices ethically.

STANDARD 8. CULTURALLY CONGRUENT PRACTICE: The IDD registered nurse engages in practice that is congruent with cultural diversity and inclusion principles, specifically as related to healthcare consumers with IDD and their families or legal guardians.

STANDARD 9. COMMUNICATION: The IDD registered nurse communicates effectively in a variety of formats in all areas of practice.

STANDARD 10. COLLABORATION: The IDD registered nurse engages in shared decision-making with healthcare consumers with IDD, their families or legal guardians, and other key stakeholders while engaging in nursing practice.

STANDARD 11. LEADERSHIP: The IDD registered nurse demonstrates leadership in professional practice settings and the profession.

STANDARD 12. EDUCATION: The IDD registered nurse acquires knowledge and attains competence that reflects current nursing practice and promotes futuristic thinking.

STANDARD 13. EVIDENCE-BASED PRACTICE AND RESEARCH: The IDD registered nurse IDD integrates relevant and current evidence and research findings into practice.

STANDARD 14. QUALITY OF PRACTICE: The IDD registered nurse contributes to quality nursing practice.

STANDARD 15. PROFESSIONAL PRACTICE EVALUATION: The IDD registered nurse evaluates one's own and others' nursing practice.

STANDARD 16. RESOURCE UTILIZATION: The IDD registered nurse utilizes appropriate resources to plan, provide, and sustain evidence-based nursing services that are safe, effective, and fiscally responsible.

STANDARD 17. ENVIRONMENTAL HEALTH: The IDD registered nurse practices in an environmentally safe and healthy manner that promotes environmentally safe settings that are beneficial to the health and well-being of individuals with IDD.

The Function of Competencies in IDD Nursing Standards

The competencies accompanying each standard may be evidence of the IDD nurse's demonstrated compliance with the corresponding standard; however, this list of competencies is not exhaustive. The application of a particular standard or competency depends on the circumstances (ANA, 2015a).

WHAT IS IDD NURSING?

IDD nursing is based on the definition of nursing, which includes

> the protection, promotion, and optimization of health and abilities, prevention of illness and injury, facilitation of healing, alleviation of suffering through the diagnosis and treatment of human response, and advocacy in the care of individuals, families, groups, communities, and populations. (ANA, 2015a, p. 11)

IDD nursing focuses on protecting, promoting, and optimizing the health and functioning ability of persons with IDD; diagnosing and treating persons with IDD to maximize quality of life and alleviate discomfort and suffering; and advocating for and with persons with IDD and their families within and across groups, communities, and society.

The integration of the art and science of nursing is described in the following detailed scope and standards of practice content. IDD nurses possess a strong foundation of knowledge and skills related to the IDD diagnoses, treatments for IDD, and the provision of health care that is unique to persons with IDD across their lifetimes. Additionally, IDD nurses understand child and adult developmental patterns (typical and delayed) as individuals with IDD have a condition that interferes with their ability to experience the typical patterns of human development that affect their ability to learn and process information. The person's development may vary in terms of communication skills, ability to comprehend and reason, and their life experiences that contribute to their differing responses. Individuals with IDD may learn differently than typically developing individuals. IDD nurses adapt healthcare procedures and processes to meet the needs of persons with IDD and their families. These individuals may have a broad range of cognitive and behavioral challenges that need to be understood and treated with respect by all healthcare providers. For example, the IDD nurse helps individuals with IDD feel comfortable when they are fearful during a medical examination or procedure. This fear of being harmed is a different response compared to individuals without IDD. IDD nurses also understand behavioral challenges associated with IDD and know how to intervene appropriately so as not to escalate challenging behaviors. The IDD nurse knows when to refer to specialized services such as dental, gynecology, obstetrics, and psychology services.

IDD nurses are members of a healthcare team focused on the provision of interprofessional services that are comprehensive in scope, as individual healthcare providers alone cannot assess, manage, or evaluate the full breadth of needs of the person with IDD. As a member of the IDD team, the nurse plans and coordinates care with the individual, family, and interdisciplinary providers. These interprofessional providers include advocates, dieticians, occupational and physical therapists, primary and specialty care physicians, social workers, special educators, speech and language specialists, child life specialists, and family members who address the ongoing and long-term needs of the individual and family members. IDD nurses understand and value each profession's contribution to assessment, treatment, and evaluation of the outcomes of a person with IDD, with the family and individual at the center of any interprofessional evaluation or treatment.

Advanced advocacy skills and greater knowledge of resources are needed to ensure that persons with IDD have their health needs identified and then move toward optimal health. Values such as respect of self and others, individual dignity, and having personal choices are critical for persons with IDD to promote their access to high-quality health care. IDD nurses support individuals with the dignity of taking risks in making choices pertaining to their health and other lifestyle decisions.

The advocacy role in IDD nursing practice is essential, as individuals with IDD and their families and those who care for them can face extraordinary challenges in accessing health care and other services. IDD nurses advocate for the health and well-being of persons with IDD and encourage persons with IDD and their families to advocate in policy arenas for their health and a healthy and safe environment. IDD nurses also advocate for policies that promote healthy and safe environments that address issues such as bullying, including cyberbullying, for those with IDD.

Early federal legislation provided the foundation for subsequent federal laws enacted to more definitively address the rights and protections of individuals with disabilities, including those with IDD. The Civil Rights Act of 1964 prohibited discrimination on the basis of sex, race, color, national origin, and religion. This legislation also prohibited racial segregation in schools, employment, and public accommodations. Later, in 1977, Section 504 was added to the Rehabilitation Act of 1973. This provision, the first of its kind, prohibited discrimination of individuals with disabilities in any programs receiving federal assistance.

Policy advocacy involves understanding the legal ramifications of federal and state legislative mandates that impact not only the rights and protections of individuals with IDD and their families but also the clinical implications for care across the life course. The legislative intent of the Americans with Disabilities Act (ADA), enacted in 1990 (PL 101–336), was to provide "…a clear and comprehensive national mandate for the elimination of discrimination against individuals with disabilities" by extending equal protections and rights to them. The ADA built upon the existing legislation of the Rehabilitation Act of 1973 and the Civil Rights Act of 1964. The ADA extended civil rights protections in these five areas: employment, public services and transportation, public accommodations, telecommunications, and miscellaneous.

The Individuals with Disabilities Education Act (IDEA), first authorized in 1990 and now known as the Individuals with Disabilities Education Improvement Act (IDEIA) of 2004, created sweeping changes in the provisions of services and supports for students with disabilities, including students with IDD. This legislation addressed reforms for services across the life course from infancy to emerging adulthood at age 22 years. IDEA and subsequent authorizations identified requirements for early intervention programs for infants with and at risk for IDD that included the use of IFSPs that provided a comprehensive plan of care based upon a family-centered plan of care and the infant's needs. Other provisions enumerated the requirements for the development and implementation of Individual Education Plans (IEP) for students beginning during the preschool years to and Individual Transition Plans (ITP) beginning at age 16 or earlier, to the post-high school years of community living skills programs for emerging adults through age 22 years.

Inspired by his own family experience of having a sister with an intellectual disability, President John F. Kennedy signed into law the Mental Retardation Facilities and Community Mental Health Centers Construction Act of 1963. This legislation and subsequent reauthorizations, including the Developmental Disabilities Assistance and Bill of Rights Act Amendments of 2000, were enacted to support the development of service and support systems for persons with IDD and their families. These programs include the State Councils on Developmental Disabilities, State Protection and Advocacy Systems (P & A), and University Centers for Excellence in Developmental Disabilities (UCEDD) Education, Research, and Service.

These federal initiatives and state-level regulations provide essential rights and protections to individuals with IDD and their families. The intent of these legislative acts is designed to ensure individuals with IDD receive needed services and supports that will enable their full inclusion in community life, enable full access to educational, employment, health, and community services, and assure their legal rights and protections. It is essential that IDD nurses are knowledgeable about these laws to ensure individuals with IDD and their families have full access to needed services and supports across the life course. Additionally, it is expected that IDD nurses will provide individuals with IDD and their families with needed guidance. It is also essential that IDD nurses stay current as these and other federal or state policies change that may impact their ability to sustain the legal rights and protections for individuals with IDD and families to receive appropriate education, employment, and health services in their communities. Becoming involved with state and federal policy changes is an important component of advocacy in today's healthcare environments.

IDD nurses assess, implement, and evaluate plans that keep individuals with IDD safe and connected appropriately to medical care, health services (particularly specialty care as they transition to adult care), and resources in the community, including transportation, accessible and affordable housing, and adequate food to live life to the fullest. Other activities that foster improved quality of life include involvement in community recreational programs and in opportunities that foster socialization with age-appropriate peers as social isolation is epidemic in this population.

WHEN NURSING OCCURS

The nursing care of persons with IDD takes place in all settings in which nurses are employed. The settings in which nurses often interact with persons with IDD are in various healthcare settings, school-based settings, community-based facilities, work sites, and large regional developmental centers. The relationships between the nurse and the person with IDD often last many years.

The care of persons with IDD needs to be developed considering the history of care and future needs of the individual and should involve the person with IDD, their family or legal guardians, and an interprofessional team. For example, in early childhood and school-aged individuals, an IFSP, an IEP, or an Individualized Transition Plan (ITP) are developed in such teams. School nurses take part in developing those plans for many individuals with IDD. The membership of the team will change as the person with IDD ages or moves. It is a commitment across the person's life course to anticipate needs and problems, reduce or eliminate problems in the present time, and regularly evaluate identified needs and problems retrospectively in order to better address such needs and problems in the future. It is important that anticipatory guidance is identified and described across the life course for conditions resulting in IDD. Much is known about these conditions during the pediatric years, but less is known and documented in the literature for the adult years and at end of life.

THE HOW OF IDD NURSING

The "how" of nursing practice is defined as the ways, means, methods, processes, and manner by which the registered nurse practices professionally. The ways in which registered nurses practice reflect integration of the five core practice competencies of all healthcare professionals: healthcare consumer-centered practice, evidence-based practice, interprofessional collaboration, use of informatics, and continuous quality improvement (ANA, 2015a; IOM, 2003). Registered nurses recognize that using a holistic approach requires incorporation of all relevant data when implementing the nursing process. Such applies to the registered nurse specializing in IDD.

To achieve the best healthcare consumer outcomes, the "how" requires the registered nurse who specializes in IDD to employ evidence-based practice as a means to incorporate the best available evidence, healthcare consumer preferences, provider expertise, and contextual resources in which nursing is delivered. Closely linked to the best healthcare consumer outcomes is the need for effective interprofessional collaboration. Thus, an essential component of the "how" of registered nursing is care coordination (ANA, 2013b), requiring effective communications by all stakeholders.

Additionally, the "how" of registered nursing practice includes predictable and comprehensive communication using approaches such as informatics, electronic health records, and established system processes to prevent errors. Methods may include situation, background, assessment, and recommendation (SBAR; The Joint Commission, 2012) and evidence-based methods of teamwork and communication skill building such as TeamSTEPPS (Agency for Healthcare Research and Quality, n.d.; ANA, 2015a; Department of Defense, 2014).

Finally, the "how" of registered nursing practice reflects the manner in which the registered nurse who specializes in IDD practices according to the *Code of Ethics for Nurses with Interpretive Statements*, standards for professional nursing practice, institutional review boards' protocols, and directives of other governing and regulatory bodies that guide the conduct of professional nursing practice (ANA, 2015a). Nursing's *Social Policy Statement: The Essence of the Profession* describes professional nursing's social contract with society and includes the registered nurse and APRN who specializes in IDD nursing (ANA, 2010a, p. 6). Consult Nursing's *Social Policy Statement* (ANA, 2010a) for discussion of other contents important to understanding the societal context related to the decision-making and conduct of professional nursing practice.

INTEGRATING THE SCIENCE AND ART OF IDD NURSING

Like the profession of nursing, the nursing specialty of IDD is built on a core body of knowledge that reflects its components of science and art. Nursing in IDD requires judgment and skills based on biological, physical, behavioral, and social sciences. Nurses use critical thinking to apply the best available evidence and research data when responding to the needs of individuals with IDD, evaluating the quality and effectiveness of nursing practice, and seeking to optimize outcomes for individuals with IDD and their families or legal guardians (ANA, 2015a).

Consistent with the profession of nursing, IDD nursing promotes the delivery of holistic care that is centered on individuals with IDD and their families or legal guardians and those who care for them with the goals of achieving optimal health outcomes through the life course and across the health–illness continuum. This occurs in an environmental context that acknowledges culture, ethics, law, politics, economics, access to healthcare resources, and competing priorities. Similarly, IDD nursing promotes the health of communities by advocating for social and environmental justice, community engagement, and access to high-quality and equitable health care to maximize population health outcomes and minimize health disparities. IDD nursing advocates for the well-being, comfort, dignity, and humanity of all individuals, families, groups, communities, and populations. IDD nursing focuses on healthcare consumer and interprofessional collaboration, sharing of knowledge, scientific discovery, and social welfare.

THE ART OF IDD NURSING

Optimal health for persons with IDD requires a holistic, caring, culturally sensitive, and interprofessional approach. IDD nurses possess unique skills in their comprehensive care of persons with IDD and their families or legal guardians. These skills include sustaining long-term relationships based on trust, communicating through verbal and nonverbal avenues, handling unpredictable behavior and situations, developing plans of care that are both short- and long-term, and including a variety of individuals and disciplines in planning such care (Appelgren, Bahtsevani, Persson, & Borglin, 2018; Jaques, Lewis, O'Reilly, Wiese, & Wilson, 2018). Specifically, the IDD nurse must be able to communicate effectively with individuals with IDD who may have difficulty communicating through usual written or verbal channels and understand and interpret the signs and cues sent by individuals with IDD to communicate their needs and desires.

Because nursing includes the diagnosis and treatment of human responses to actual or potential health problems and comorbid disabilities, nurses focus on modifying the impact of illness and disease on individuals with IDD and aim to prevent further disability. When individuals with IDD have a disease and illness, IDD nurses should be careful to distinguish signs and symptoms of the disease and illness from characteristics of the disability. This is especially important when an individual's disability manifests in ways that are similar to a disease or illness. When planning and implementing care, IDD nurses may have opportunities to develop innovative and creative approaches to assure optimal and positive outcomes for the individual with IDD and his or her family or legal guardians.

Care and Caring in IDD Nursing Practice

The relationship between the IDD nurse, the person with IDD, and their family or legal guardians builds on a bond that is often long term, based on verbal and nonverbal communication and mutual respect, while recognizing strengths and helping to mitigate challenges. Nurses support the right of individuals with IDD to self-determination. That is, individuals with IDD have opportunities and experiences that enable them to have control in their lives and to advocate for themselves (AAIDD Board of Directors, The Arc of the United States [ARC] Board of Directors, & Chapters of the Arc, 2018). As self-advocates, individuals with IDD should be heard, respected, and supported to fully participate in their own health care. Nurses work to ensure that individuals with IDD and their families or legal guardians have the knowledge and skills to engage in informed decision-making about health. Family members and substitute decision-makers may need assistance in understanding the importance of self-determination and the limits that self-determination can place on their own authority to make decisions with and for the individual with IDD.

IDD nurses (a) believe in individuals with IDD and their abilities to meet developmental and life course milestones, (b) work to understand the meaning of health and health-related events from the perspective of individuals with IDD and their families or legal guardians, (c) are emotionally present for individuals with IDD and their families or legal guardians, (d) carry out health-related activities and tasks for individuals with IDD and their families or legal guardians when those persons cannot carry out those activities and tasks themselves, and (e) support and facilitate transitions and unpredictable events experienced by individuals with IDD and their families or legal guardians. IDD nursing care for persons with IDD must include age-related preventive care in addition to care for their unique health problems.

IDD nurses should be mindful that the experiences of individuals with IDD in society may be those of oppression and limitations on their ability to fully participate in their communities and be treated equally.

Health services such as routine gynecological/obstetric care, mammograms, and preventive and therapeutic dental services should be accessible to individuals with IDD. There should be a balance between undertreatment—the limitations of treatment based on IDD diagnosis—and overtreatment—the unwillingness to recognize when treatment is no longer beneficial. IDD nurses may have advocacy and educator roles in the decision-making process with the individual with IDD, if capable; the family, if appropriate; and others involved in the individual's care.

Advances in assistive and medical technology contribute to improved health, functioning ability, and quality of life in individuals with IDD. Assistive technology (AT) should benefit individuals with IDD by improving independence, mobility, communication, and ability to control their environments (AAIDD, Arc, & Chapters of The Arc, 2018). Medical technology should be directed toward improving their quality of life and relieving pain, isolation, fear, and physical discomforts. Individuals with IDD should be provided with information and assistance to comprehend that information, for example, about treatment, services, and technology offered to them. They should also have the opportunity to accept or refuse what is offered. When information cannot be provided in a way that takes into account the communication and cognitive challenges of the individual with IDD to ensure informed consent, then the individual's advocate (i.e., legal guardians, healthcare power of attorney, or surrogate decision-maker) should be involved to assure that the individual's demonstrations of acceptance or refusal are respected and followed (AAIDD, Arc, and Chapters of The Arc, 2018; Vanderbilt Kennedy Center for Excellence in Developmental Disabilities, 2018). Nurses should advocate for a careful evaluation of the benefits and risks of a proposed treatment for an individual with or at risk for IDD and not accept a categorical denial or plan to institute treatment based on another's estimation of the quality of life of the individual with or at risk for IDD.

Genetic and genomic advances promise both gains for and threats to individuals with IDD. Sometime in the future, the basis for IDD may be identified and eventually "treated" with gene therapy. If this technology evolves, there may be social pressure to submit to the treatment to ameliorate or eliminate the disability, and even less tolerance for the spectrum of human difference. Some assume that if a prenatal disability is detected, the mother (or parents) will choose to terminate the pregnancy. IDD nurses respect the autonomous decisions of the mother but also grant that the mother's decision may be influenced by society's response to individuals with IDD and tolerance for difference.

The IDD nurse must have advanced assessment skills to correctly identify issues related to the health and safety of the individual with IDD, including all forms of bullying (i.e., bullying associated with school or community or cyberbullying), chronological and mental age development in all domains, social relationships, and activities of daily living (ADL). Such assessments are used for short- and long-term care planning and implementation, regular evaluations, and consequent adjustments. Creativity, adaptations, patience, and involvement from the individual with IDD, their family or legal guardians, and other disciplines are required for optimal outcomes.

It is also important to note that nurses who specialize in this population are often stigmatized themselves. Such misunderstanding comes from other nurses not involved in this specialty and even other professionals in the field. Having a network of nurses working in the field through formal and informal means is helpful for support and consultative input on difficult care situations.

Cultural Components of Care

The nurse provides care to individuals with IDD and their families or legal guardians and those who care for them in a manner that reflects sensitivity to culture and varied expressions of care among all forms and types of cultures (Leininger, 1988) and supports the implementation of caring processes built on Watson's framework (2012, 2008, 1999). Persons with IDD are a minority culture in which positive and negative behaviors and opinions are found by other persons and cultures, and these have existed across time. Our understanding of cultural literacy must go beyond race and encompass all forms of culture, including persons with IDD.

THE SCIENCE OF IDD NURSING

Both qualitative and quantitative research has been conducted to identify and describe conditions resulting in IDD, to detail best practices in the treatment of primary and comorbid conditions across the life course, and to develop policy and procedures for optimal care of persons with IDD. Nurses have been involved in such research over the years through their own original studies as well as the translation of research findings in their practice.

IDD Nursing Knowledge

IDD nursing knowledge is best described through a historical perspective. This section provides a summary of the history of education of nurses and nursing care in this specialty.

Asylums, institutions, and hospital-based nursing schools were the first to provide education for nurses who specialized in the care of persons of any age who had IDD; however, the term IDD was not used until the mid-20th century. Until the early 20th century, persons with IDD were diagnosed as having mental illness, and their care took place in settings where persons with all forms of mental illness were housed. After WWI, an improved understanding of mental illness emerged, and the care of persons with IDD as we now know it was more specifically detailed. Offensive terminology was often used at that time to describe individuals with IDD.

In the early 1960s, President Kennedy brought needed attention to the living conditions of persons of all ages with IDD, then called *mental retardation*. New legislation was introduced, and for the first time, funding became available for this population. Large institutional settings remained the primary place of residence for persons of all ages with IDD until the late 1960s. It was the social norm to place newborns and children with known conditions resulting in IDD in institutions as soon as possible so as not to burden families, either financially or through social stigma.

After public attention to the custodial and often inhumane care of persons with IDD in the early 1970s, radical changes took place. Many individuals with IDD were moved back to their homes and to newly formed community settings, such as group homes, semi-independent living arrangements, and smaller congregate settings (e.g., 16 beds). The transition from institutional to community living settings continues with state by state variation.

Today, newborns with IDD are no longer placed in institutional settings. Most individuals with IDD live with their families in the community. Others live in small-group community settings. Only the most severely affected individuals who require substantial medical care remain in larger developmental centers (Nehring, 1999; Nehring & Lindsey, 2016).

IDD nursing care has also evolved through time. Early documentation about nursing care was written either by physicians or nurses who cared for both persons with IDD and mental illness. Literature by nurses about the nursing care of persons with IDD first appeared with any frequency in the 1950s. At that time, nurses in institutional settings did little more than give medications and record vital signs and occasional weight measurements. Some public health nurses provided care for children with IDD who remained at home; however, parents were often encouraged to place their children in institutions by the time they reached school age.

The first national meeting for nurses specializing in the care of children with IDD was sponsored by the Children's Bureau in 1958 (Nehring, 2010). In the 1960s, nursing care in the institution resembled nursing care provided in hospitals. The role of the nurse expanded to include education and research. APRNs were employed by some institutions, and post-baccalaureate and graduate programs emerged to provide education designed especially for the care of children and adolescents with IDD. Interdisciplinary faculty (including nurses) at University-Affiliated Programs and Facilities (UAPs or UAFs) established by President Kennedy in universities across the country, offered interdisciplinary education to future specialists (including nurses) in the field; conducted research on topics related to mental retardation; and provided health and social services to individuals with IDD and their families.

In the 1960s, nurses began to write more prolifically about the care of children with IDD conditions. The increased numbers of articles and books, some of which are now considered classics, were especially useful for public health nurses. Developmental diagnostic clinics were established across the country to identify and refer children with IDD for developmental and health care when appropriate. Nursing consultants who specialized in this field were hired by the Children's Bureau; Division of Neurological Diseases and Stroke, U.S. Public Health Service; Mental Retardation Division, Department of Health, Education, and Welfare; Association of Retarded Children; and the United Cerebral Palsy Associations, Inc. National meetings were convened for these nursing specialists, and the first standards of nursing practice for this specialty emerged in 1968, *The Guidelines for Nursing Standards in Residential Centers for the Mentally Retarded* (Haynes, 1968; Nehring, 1999, 2010).

The 1970s saw the first national education legislation, mandating that all children with IDD receive a free and appropriate public education from the ages of 3 through 21 years. During that period, school nurses sought education and resources about IDD nursing and roles for school nurses who work with students with IDD and students with special healthcare needs. Advanced practice roles for nurses in the IDD specialty continued to expand, including roles in schools and early intervention programs for the infant from birth to three years of age.

Publications and regular national and regional meetings about IDD nursing continued throughout the 1970s. Special IDD nursing courses also began to appear in nursing programs across the country (Hahn, 2003; Nehring, 1999, 2010). Legislation (P.L. 91–517) passed in October 1970 during President Nixon's administration changed the terms "mental retardation" to "developmental disabilities" and "clinical training" to "interdisciplinary training." The definition of developmental disabilities was broadened in the Developmentally Disabled Assistance and Bill of Rights Act (P.L. 94–103), which was signed into law by President Gerald Ford in 1975. In addition to mental retardation, the new definition of developmental disabilities included cerebral palsy, epilepsy, autism, and dyslexia if it resulted from one of those other disabilities. As part of that legislation, a national task force was convened, which modified the definition of developmental disabilities in 1977 to eliminate references to specific conditions and to emphasize substantial functional limitations or "impairment" (Thompson & O'Quinn, 1979).

Interdisciplinary care was the norm in the 1980s when all disciplines worked together with individuals and family members of those with IDD to assess and plan care in a variety of settings (Nehring, 1999; Nehring & Lindsey, 2016). In 1980, ANA published *School Nurses Working with Handicapped Children* (Igoe et al., 1980). Later in the 1980s, two sets of standards of nursing practice for nurses specializing in this field emerged: *Standards of Nursing Practice in Mental Retardation/Developmental Disabilities* (Aggen & Moore, 1984) and *Standards for the Clinical Advanced Practice Registered Nurse in Developmental Disabilities/Handicapping Conditions* (Austin, Challela, Huber, Sciarillo, & Stade, 1987).

Emphasis on the adult with IDD emerged in the nursing literature in the 1990s. An examination of the individual with IDD across the life course was first highlighted in *A Life-Span Approach to Nursing Care for Individuals with Developmental Disabilities* (Roth & Morse, 1994). Nursing standards for this field were also revised: *Standards of Developmental Disabilities Nursing Practice* (Aggen, DeGennaro, Fox, Hahn, Logan, & VonFumetti, 1995) and *Statement on the Scope and Standards for the Nurse Who Specializes in Developmental Disabilities and/or Mental Retardation* (Nursing Division of the American Association on Mental Retardation and American Nurses Association [ANA], 1998). Other related standards of nursing practice in early intervention (ANA Consensus Committee, 1993), care of children and adolescents with special health and developmental needs (ANA Consensus Committee, 1994), and genetics (ISONG & ANA, 1998) were issued as well.

In the first years of the 21st century, a greater effort was made to provide educational materials for nursing students and nurses in practice who care for persons of all ages with IDD (Betz & Sawin, 2018; Hahn, 2003; Nehring, 2005). In 2010, a comprehensive text on IDD nursing was published based upon a life course approach entitled, *Nursing Care for Individuals with Developmental Disabilities: An Integrated Approach* (Betz & Nehring, 2010). However, IDD nursing remains an area where nursing students, in general, receive little information about or clinical experience with persons who have IDD. Concentrated efforts by nursing experts in the field and national organizations, such as AAIDD and DDNA, to establish standards for IDD nursing education, should persist.

This specialty field of nursing has changed greatly from its early years. As the healthcare system continues to evolve, so will the nursing care of persons with IDD of all ages. Such care continues to occur in a variety of settings and at both the professional registered nurse and APRN levels. Continued publication and research into such nursing care are needed, as are additional didactic and clinical content materials for nursing students.

Research in IDD Nursing

Nurses have faced a myriad of challenges in researching the IDD population over the years that include societal changes, laws affecting education, Institutional Review Board approvals for this vulnerable population, and research expertise in those nurses working in the field. These factors have resulted in difficulty in obtaining data for the development of evidence-based IDD nursing interventions. There is clearly a need for consistent nursing education, nursing management, and more research in the field of IDD nursing (Auberry, 2018).

There have been champions of IDD health care who have accomplished research in the field, which IDD nurses can use as a basis for future research. Dorothea Dix is thought to be the first leader in IDD nursing. Although Dix was not a nurse, she is viewed by many as being instrumental in the development of IDD, public health, and mental health nursing (Nehring, 1999). Using her careful observations of the living conditions of individuals with IDD, Dix made many appeals for more hygienic buildings for individuals with IDD and mental illness, and some of her efforts met with success (Dix, 1847). For example, she spoke to the Massachusetts legislature in 1843 about the conditions of jails, asylums, and almshouses in Massachusetts (Dix, 1976). Consistent with Florence Nightingale's call for nurses to use their observations to bring about change (Nightingale, 1859), Dix used her observations to inform and influence legislators to improve the living conditions of individuals with IDD (Nehring, 1999, 2010).

In the 1960s, nurses began conducting and publishing their research about individuals with IDD. These early nurse researchers relied on models, research findings, and research methods from the fields of education, medicine, physical therapy, cognitive and developmental psychology, psychiatry, public health, speech therapy, and sociology. Miller (1979) described a program that was implemented from 1962 through 1964 to teach personnel in the Central Wisconsin Colony and Training School to provide speech and physical therapy to residents. Pat McNelly (1966) conducted a study that "was a precursor to the development of the transdisciplinary model of care delivery" (Nehring, 1999, p. 79). A cross-disciplinary project, the Mimosa Project, was funded to teach adolescent girls with IDD daily living skills (Devine, 1983). Barclay, Goulet, Holtgrewe, and Sharp (1962) examined parents' evaluations of the clinic services provided to their children with IDD. By 1970, many studies related to IDD had been or were being carried out by nurses, and graduate students in nursing programs were focusing their dissertation research on IDD. Between 1970 and 2019, more than 200 nursing dissertations related to IDD were completed.

Nurses contribute to research and scholarly work related to IDD across the life course. Two nurses who are well recognized for their work in developmental disabilities focused their work on infants and children with or at risk for IDD. Una H. Haynes, a committed nurse who made many contributions to the field of developmental disabilities, was on the national staff team of the United Cerebral Palsy Associations, Inc., and is credited with developing the transdisciplinary approach to early intervention for infants with developmental disabilities (Haynes, 1974). Kathryn Barnard began her work with children with IDD (Barnard, 1966, 1968). She developed the Nursing Child Assessment Satellite Training (now referred to as the Parent-Child Relationship Programs at the Barnard Center) and was an advocate for prevention in nursing and mental health. A third nurse, Cecily Betz, has dedicated her life work to the conceptual understanding of transitions in care for persons with IDD (e.g., Betz, Nehring, & Lobo, 2015; Mahan, Betz, Okumura, & Ferris, 2017). While there is clearly a need for focused research on the myriad of related concepts to the field of IDD in the future, there are ongoing efforts to marry research on general aspects of nursing practice related to caring for families and individuals to include special needs populations that are inclusive of IDD including autism and behavioral health, or research that transects concepts such as family management, support, and family-centered care (Christian, 2018; Ford et al., 2018).

Evidence-Based Practice in IDD Nursing

Just as nursing research has evolved and developed across the profession, nursing research in IDD has evolved and continues its development, including an emphasis on evidence-based practice. Quantitative, qualitative, and mixed-methods studies are conducted across the life course using nursing and non-nursing theories. Nurses working in the field of IDD have long recognized the importance of interprofessional collaboration in practice. Likewise, interprofessional collaboration is essential for many nursing research activities, including the identification and implementation of evidence-based practice related to IDD.

Nurse researchers have focused their research on specific conditions that result in or are associated with IDD, roles and responsibilities of nurses working in this field, families or legal guardians and family-centered care, and education of nurses and others about IDD. Nehring (1999) called for research that (a) evaluates programs and services provided to individuals with IDD; (b) examines adult health care, adult development, and the educational needs of caregivers across the life course of individuals with IDD; (c) explores issues related to genetics; and (d) explores the perspectives of individuals with IDD and their families or legal guardians and those that care for them that need to be addressed by nurses. Such research remains consistent, as Betz and Sawin (2018) echoed these research needs and added better understanding of and improved practice models for care coordination across the life course. Furthermore, efforts are being made to include consumers and families as members of the research project to provide input as to the development of the research question/issue to be investigated, methods for recruitment, and other aspects. In addition, new challenges related to the complexities of health care and demands for healthcare reform also require attention. For example, NASN has published evidence-based position statements related to children with special healthcare needs (e.g., *Chronic Health Conditions [Students with]: The Role of the School Nurse*, 2017a; *The Role of the 21st*

Century School Nurse, 2018; and *Transition Planning for Students with Chronic Health Conditions,* 2019a).

Nurse researchers should examine nursing practice in IDD to demonstrate that staffing is adequate to ensure quality care for individuals with IDD and their families or legal guardians. Consistent with the call for continual evaluation of nursing practice, as stated in *The Code of Ethics for Nurses with Interpretive Statements* (ANA, 2015b), ongoing evaluation of patient outcomes and learning needs of nurses working with individuals with IDD and their families or legal guardians, and dissemination of information to address these outcomes and needs, are critical.

THE WHERE OF IDD NURSING PRACTICE

Nurses care for persons of all ages with IDD in any environment and setting in which nurses practice. A few salient examples follow to illustrate the breadth of settings and environments in which nurses specializing in IDD nursing practice. By the 1950s, many infants born with an intellectual or developmental disability were institutionalized. Many times, the mother was told that her newborn had died since she was unconscious during birth, and the father signed away the parental rights and kept the secret. With deinstitutionalization and federal and state law changes beginning in the 1960s and 1970s, more infants and children with IDD went home after birth, remained at home with their families, and were able to attend school. Today, residential institutions specifically for those with IDD still exist in some states, although those numbers are decreasing. Some communities have developmental centers to support individuals with IDD, which may be age focused, for example, for early childhood, school age, or adults with IDD. Supports for individuals with IDD are also provided through home health care, school-based care, postacute care, assisted living and long-term care facilities, and community-based living, faith communities, outpatient, and ambulatory settings are standard settings for care, yet developmental centers for individuals with severe IDD still exist. The care of persons with IDD in each of these settings requires the services of nurses. This evolution has greater importance as transitions in care, cost reduction measures, financial penalties for adverse outcomes, and healthcare reform initiatives materialize.

School nursing is an example of a nursing discipline in which nurses spend a great deal of time with individuals with IDD. According to the National Association of Elementary School Principals (Wherry, 2004), the average child spends about six hours a day at school for 180 school days a year. School nurses are often closely involved with children and youth with an IDD since they may have chronic health problems or other issues. In addition, school nurses are often likely to work with their parents or guardians, teachers, and other school staff. School nurses use the nursing process to develop nursing care plans and emergency plans in conjunction with children's parents and healthcare providers. They also teach students, parents, and staff about care. They often participate in multidisciplinary teams that develop IFSPs, IEPs, and ITPs for children and youth with IDD and advocate for students in schools and communities (Bargeron, Contri, Gibbons, Ruch-Ross, & Sanabria, 2015; Quinn & Smolinski, 2017; Singer, 2013).

In addition to the setting noted above, nurses specializing in IDD may be employed in colleges and universities as faculty or practicing nurses, nurse practitioners, or administrators of nurse-managed clinics or school health centers, which are clinical settings associated with schools. There is a scarcity of nursing faculty and scholars with IDD as their area of expertise and scholarship focus. When present, they are often employed at universities that are designated as University Centers of Excellence in Developmental Disabilities (UCEDD).

Technological advances for persons with IDD have allowed them to live more integrated lives and provide another area where nurses can use entrepreneurial skills in new roles. Nurses often play active roles in accessing needed technology for their patients, adapting it for their optimal use, evaluating it for continued use, and developing their own ideas for use by persons with IDD.

The IDD nurse plays an active advocacy role in the facilitation of full integration of persons with IDD into all aspects of community and residential settings to achieve their optimal level of functioning. Advocacy and a commitment to community integration with optimal individual functioning are key characteristics of nurses working on behalf of people with IDD and their families or legal guardians and those that care for them. From advocacy with legislatures at the state and national levels to individual advocacy supporting choice and self-determination for the individual with IDD, nurses in the specialty are passionate about the population and about achieving social justice for them. Assisting an individual with IDD to transition from supported health care (e.g., practicing medication administration) in high school to supported health care in a community work setting or from living in an institutional setting into a less restrictive setting, such as their own home or a supervised apartment or group home; to obtain quality health care, identifying and responding to allegations of abuse; and aiding in healthcare decision-making by supporting the individual or identifying a surrogate are all crucial areas for advocacy intervention.

Though there are many challenges in the care of persons of all ages with IDD, such as communication difficulties, multiple comorbid conditions, public ignorance, and societal prejudice, there are also many rewards. Learning about and working with this population, for whom significant health disparities have only recently been identified, can enlighten and add meaning to nursing practice and personal life. Nurses learn to appreciate individual strengths and assist individuals with IDD to live full lives and participate fully in caring for their preventive and specific health needs.

Healthy Work Environments for Nursing Practice

Characteristics of IDD Nursing Practice Tenet #5 explicitly state that "a strong link exists between professional work environment and the IDD registered nurse's ability to provide quality health care and achieve optimal outcomes" (Nehring et al., 2013). The *Nursing: Scope and Standards of Practice,* 3rd Edition, states that "all must be mindful of the health and safety of both the healthcare consumer and the healthcare worker in any setting, providing a sense of safety, respect, and empowerment to and for all persons" (2015, p. 27). Several models of healthy work environments have been recognized and supported by ANA. These models are universal and can be adapted to IDD nursing practice.

Safe Patient Handling and Mobility (SPHM)

Individuals with IDD possess various levels of thinking, reasoning, planning, and problem solving, placing them at greater risk for safety issues. IDD nurses must be equipped to identify and manage potential harmful situations for both the individual with IDD and the nursing staff. Safe patient handling begins with trust and communication appropriate to the level of the patient with IDD or the caregiver. This is especially crucial when individuals with IDD become even more vulnerable when hospitalized or removed from a familiar setting. A sample Toolkit for Primary Care Providers on communicating effectively with individual's with IDD is available at www.iddtoolkit.vkcsites.org/general-issues/communicating-effectively/. IDD nurses should also be trained in responding to and reporting abuse that so often occurs among people with IDD, especially women and children (Byrne, 2018). Additionally, aggressive behavior toward staff is a concern.

In 2013, ANA, along with other professional organizations, established eight Evidence-Based Standards for Safe Patient Handling and Mobility to be used in any healthcare setting, including residential living where many individuals with IDD may reside. While these apply to the general population, they can and should be adapted to nurses caring for individuals with IDD.

1. Establishing a culture of safety, which includes ensuring safe levels of staffing, creating a nonpunitive environment, and developing a system for communication and collaboration. For example, patients with IDD may require the use of auxiliary communication aids/services such as:
    - Sign language interpreters;
    - Braille materials;
    - Simplified language documents;
    - Computer-Assisted Real Time text (CART); and
    - Large print documents.
2. Implementing and sustaining a safe patient handling and mobility program specific to the needs of the individual with IDD and their caregiver. Persons with IDD may have mobility impairments

requiring the use of wheelchairs or other assistive devices for ambulation. Issues related to mobility restrictions include: performing transfers with appropriate body mechanics and equipment; ensuring wheelchairs and ambulation devices are in good working order; and assessing the needs for durable medical equipment such as commodes, lifts, and bathing chairs/benches.

3. Incorporating ergonomic design principles to provide a safe environment of care. The IDD nurse may assess the safety of the living conditions of the individual with IDD. For instance, if the individual with IDD is a wheelchair user, the IDD nurse will ensure clear floor access to all areas of the living quarters (to prevent accidents) and will teach family members and caregivers how to assess for this safety measure.

4. Selecting, installing, and maintaining safe patient handling technology. The IDD nurse will work with the individual with IDD, family members, caregivers, and other healthcare professionals to carefully identify the individual's mobility strengths and limitations to select the technology that promotes independence and self-care safely and respectfully. Equipment and technology are adjusted as the individual's abilities change.

5. Establishing a system for education, training, and maintaining competence. Working with family members, caregivers, and the individual with IDD, the IDD nurse develops an educational plan to ensure they are properly trained on the consumer's safe handling and mobility program. The IDD nurse conducts routine training with the consumer, family members, and caregivers and modifies the program based on the consumer's needs and the environment.

6. Integrating patient-centered assessment, care planning, and technology. The degree to which the handling and mobility program meets the consumer's needs and is appropriate for the consumer's environment and living conditions should be assessed routinely. Particular attention should be given to the possible need for alteration in the program when the individual with IDD experiences challenges with behavior, health, and mobility.

7. Including safe patient handling in reasonable accommodations and post injury return to work policies. The IDD nurse strives to create an environment in which the consumer's independence is supported safely, given the resources available to the consumer, family members, caregivers, and the nurse. Resources may include communication services, staff, structural characteristics of the consumer's living environment, and family member and caregiver knowledge and ability.
8. Establishing a comprehensive evaluation system. The IDD nurse will develop a comprehensive system for routinely evaluating the extent to which the safe handling and mobility program meets the needs of the consumer, the family members or caregivers, and the staff. This evaluation will consider the consumer's health; changes in the consumer's ability; effectiveness of the existing plan to meet the needs of the individual with IDD, family members, caregivers, and staff; and the consumer's living environment.

Fatigue in Nursing Practice

IDD nurses have a responsibility to maintain their own health and well-being in order to perform at their highest level of competence. In 2017, ANA launched the Healthy Nurse Healthy Nation campaign that promotes nutrition, stress control, sleep health, and fatigue prevention (ANA, 2017). In 2017, the American Academy of Nursing released a position statement entitled Reducing Fatigue Associated with Sleep Deficiency and Work Hours in Nurses that included the following recommended actions (Caruso et al., 2017, p. 767):

- Urge nurses and employers of healthcare organizations to educate themselves about the health risks linked to shift work and long work hours and the evidence-based strategies to reduce those risks.
- Urge employers of healthcare organizations to incorporate evidence-based practices in the design of their employees' work schedules and establish policies, programs, practices, and systems at work that promote sleep health and an alert workforce.

- Urge employers to promote a workplace culture that promotes sleep health to achieve optimum functioning, health, safety, and sense of well-being of their workforce.
- Encourage employers to recognize the role of shift work, long shifts, and nurse fatigue on turnover, absenteeism, patient safety, and related costs.
- Urge experts to develop additional continuing education courses for nurses and nursing managers that relay evidence-based personal practices and workplace interventions to maximize sleep health and alertness in nurses.
- IDD nurses have an ethical responsibility to take these actions, as well as report to work alert, well-rested, and prepared to give safe, quality patient care (ANA, 2014a; ANA, 2015b).

Workplace Violence and Incivility

Healthcare workers and healthcare support personnel experience a higher amount of serious workplace violence than other private industries averaging 7.8 cases per 10,000 full-time employees in 2013 (U.S. Department of Labor, Occupational Safety and Health Administration [OSHA], 2015). This is almost 400 percent more cases than other sectors of industry, including manufacturing, construction, and retail. Workplace violence, bullying, and incivility may come from clients, coworkers, administration, and support personnel, and it is believed to be vastly under-reported (OSHA, 2015). Risk factors include: (a) working with people who have a history of violence; (b) working alone; (c) poor environmental design; (d) lack of means for communicating an incident or emergency; (e) lack of training and policies, (f) understaffing, high turnover rate; (g) working in high crime areas; (h) lifting, moving, and transporting clients; (i) lack of funding for mental health services; (j) the perception that violence is tolerated; and, (k) a fear of repercussions for reporting (OSHA, 2015).

Those who work with clients with IDD may also experience issues with role ambiguity, poor social support, and poor organization of work settings, which may lead to workplace bullying and incivility (Figueiredo-Ferraz, Grau-Alberola, Gil-Monte, & García-Juesas, 2012). Additionally, many caregivers consider that violence may be a part of the job because injuries caused by clients are often unintentional (OSHA, 2015).

Prevention of workplace violence and incivility includes identifying the risk factors specific to the work environment and developing strategies to reduce the incidence of the violence. Nurses, including nurses who specialize in IDD, must advocate for safe work environments, training, and policies that address workplace violence, bullying, and incivility (ANA, 2015a).

OPTIMAL STAFFING

Nurses working with clients with IDD practice in a variety of settings, including community settings, homes (family, individual, and group), long-term care facilities, outpatient and ambulatory settings, psychiatric and rehabilitation facilities, faith-based communities, home health, correctional facilities, assisted living homes, schools, and hospitals. Optimal staffing should be based on client needs and should support individuals with IDD to function to their full potential in a safe, efficient, and meaningful way (Bigby & Beadle-Brown, 2018). Staffing should accommodate the client's physical, emotional, spiritual, and social needs and allow for self-determination, empowerment, and community. IDD nurses should advocate for safe staffing models that support team-based care and consider principles that improve work environments and improve outcomes of clinical care (ANA, 2015a).

ANA's Principles of Nurse Staffing (2019) includes a framework to assist nurses in considering principles related to healthcare consumers, registered nurses and other staff, organization and workplace culture, the practice environment, and staffing evaluation in order to provide optimal staffing. Staff levels should reflect careful planning according to client complexity and acuity, professional nurse and staff expertise, the physical layout, and the availability of resources and technical support (Kane, Shamilyan, Mueller, Duvall, & Wilt, 2007; Needleman, 2015). IDD nurses must advocate for a culture of safety. When work environments do not promote safety and health as a priority, employees will not be able to provide error-free care (OSHA, 2015). Unhealthy work environments also lead to higher rates of staff absenteeism, higher turnover rates, and burnout.

Supports for Healthy Work Environments

ANA supports the following models of healthy work environment design. These concepts apply to the healthy work environments of IDD nursing practice as well.

AMERICAN NURSES ASSOCIATION

The initial ANA Healthy Nurse™ framework began in 2009. The definition and constructs are as follows: ANA defines the healthy nurse as:

> …one who actively focuses on creating and maintaining a balance and synergy of physical, intellectual, emotional, social, spiritual, personal, and professional well-being. Healthy nurses live life to the fullest capacity, across the wellness–illness continuum, as they become stronger role models, advocates, and educators, personally, for their families, their communities and work environments, and ultimately for their patients (ANA, 2013d).

The five Healthy Nurse™ constructs include:

- Calling to Care: Caring is the interpersonal, compassionate offering of self by which the healthy IDD nurse builds relationships with IDD patients and their families while helping them meet their physical, emotional, and spiritual goals, for all ages, in all healthcare settings, across the care continuum.
- Priority to Self-Care: Self-care and supportive environments enable the healthy IDD nurse to increase the ability to effectively manage the physical and emotional stressors of the work and home environments.
- Opportunity to Role Model: The healthy IDD nurse confidently recognizes and identifies personal health challenges in themselves and their IDD patients and families or legal guardians, thereby enabling them and their IDD patients to overcome the challenge in a collaborative, nonaccusatory manner.
- Responsibility to Educate: Using nonjudgmental approaches, considering adult learning patterns and readiness to change, the healthy IDD nurse empowers themselves and others by sharing

health, safety, wellness knowledge, skills, resources, and attitudes.
- Authority to Advocate: The healthy IDD nurse is empowered to advocate on numerous levels, including personally, interpersonally, within the work environment and the community, and at the local, state, and national levels in IDD policy development and advocacy.

The *Nursing: Scope and Standards of Practice* 3rd Edition (2015a) states that "all must be mindful of the health and safety of both the healthcare consumer and the healthcare worker in any setting, providing a sense of safety, respect, and empowerment to and for all persons" (p. 27). Several models of healthy work environments have been recognized and supported by ANA. These models are universal and can be adapted to IDD nursing practice.

AMERICAN ASSOCIATION OF CRITICAL CARE NURSES STANDARDS

Seminal work by the American Association of Critical Care Nurses (AACN) has identified six standards that must be in place to establish and maintain healthy work environments (AACN, 2016):

- Skilled Communication: Nurses must be as proficient in communication skills as they are in clinical skills.
- True Collaboration: Nurses must be relentless in pursuing and fostering true collaboration.
- Effective Decision-Making: Nurses must be valued and committed partners in making policy, directing and evaluating clinical care, and leading organizational operations.
- Appropriate Staffing: Staffing must ensure the effective match between patient needs and nurse competencies.
- Meaningful Recognition: Nurses must be recognized and must recognize others for the value each brings to the work of the organization.
- Authentic Leadership: Nurse leaders must fully embrace the imperative of a healthy work environment, authentically live it, and engage others in its achievements.

The environments where IDD nurses' practice are varied and complex. Yet these six standards can be universally applied. A quality healthcare environment can be achieved by aligning IDD nurse competencies to patient needs within the context of these six standards.

HIGH-PERFORMING INTERPROFESSIONAL TEAMS

Individuals with IDD often have complex and chronic conditions requiring team collaboration among healthcare professionals and family members. IDD registered nurses are experts at person-centered care, an approach that places the person with an IDD at the center of the team. IDD registered nurses are role models who consider the individual with IDD's values, desires, family system, and goals while engaging with other members of the interprofessional team.

The Interprofessional Education Collaborative Expert Panel ([IECEP], 2011) introduced four core competencies of collaborative practice that can be applied to all settings where IDD registered nurses practice. Teams must be educated, prepared, and committed to addressing the ethical issues among people with IDD, including higher rates of poverty and victimization, lack of access to care, and educational and employment opportunities.

1. Values and Ethics: Work with Individuals of other professions to maintain a climate of mutual respect and shared values (IECEP, p. 19). Most often IDD nurses are team members that collaboratively assess, plan, implement, and evaluate interdisciplinary plans of care for individuals with IDD in a variety of settings. Effective interdisciplinary collaboration requires an understanding of and respect for the discipline-specific scope of practice of each team member that is needed for the care of individuals with IDD.
2. Roles and Responsibilities: Use the knowledge of one's own role and those of other professions to assess and address the healthcare needs of the patients and populations served (IECEP, p. 21). Interdisciplinary care is most effective when discipline-specific

team members understand the scope of practice and roles that each member contributes to the care environments of individuals with IDD.
3. Interprofessional Communication: Communicate with patients, families, communities, and other health professionals in a responsive and responsible manner that supports a team approach to health maintenance and the treatment of disease (IECEP, p. 23). Communication is most effective when the interdisciplinary team designates a team coordinator to serve as the primary liaison of communication to the patient, family, and others. A team coordinator serves as the communication conduit of the team members to ensure a specified and single source for communication is available to the patient, family, and others and that the communication is clear, accurate, and responsive.
4. Teams and Teamwork: Apply relationship-building values and the principles of team dynamics to perform effectively in different team roles to plan and deliver patient- and population-centered care that is safe, timely, efficient, effective, and equitable (IECEP, p. 25). Adherence to these competencies will not only improve health outcomes of persons with IDD but may alleviate professional burnout of IDD nurses.

KEY INFLUENCES ON THE QUALITY AND ENVIRONMENT OF NURSING PRACTICE

The field of IDD nursing faces several distinct challenges. These challenges include: complexity of care, educational preparation specific to the field is lacking, role ambiguity exists across varied practice settings, and a scarcity of evidence-based research to guide practice (Auberry, 2018). IDD registered nurses not only need to be aware of these challenges but should take the lead in removing barriers that prevent a productive, high-quality environment within which to practice.

The healthcare industry, legislation, and regulatory bodies are major external influences on the work environment of all nurses. IDD registered nurses must keep abreast of trends and changes to healthcare delivery;

they must practice to the full extent of their education. IDD registered nurses can ensure that their consumers have access to high-quality health care thus alleviating disparities among people with IDD (ANA, 2015a; IOM, 2011). Two important documents that IDD nurses should be aware of are "The Future of Disability in America, IOM Report" (2007) and Healthy People 2030: People with Disabilities (Office of Disease Prevention and Health Promotion, Office of the Assistant Secretary for Health, Office of the Secretary, & U.S. Department of Health and Human Services, 2020).

SOCIETAL, CULTURAL, AND ETHICAL DIMENSIONS DESCRIBE THE WHY AND HOW OF IDD NURSING

IDD nursing is responsive to the changing needs of society that include its changing diversity, the legislative changes, and the expanding knowledge base of its theoretical and scientific domains. One objective of nurses who specialize in IDD is to achieve positive outcomes that maximize quality of life from the time of diagnosis across the entire life course. Registered nurses specializing in IDD facilitate the interprofessional, comprehensive, and cultural care provided by healthcare professionals, paraprofessionals, and volunteers. In other instances, IDD registered nurses consult with other colleagues to inform decision-making and planning to meet the healthcare needs of individuals with IDD. Registered nurses specializing in IDD participate in interprofessional teams in which the overlapping skills complement and enhance each member's individual efforts.

IDD nursing practice, like all nursing practice, is fundamentally an independent practice in that registered nurses are accountable for nursing judgments made and actions taken in the course of their nursing practice. Therefore, the registered nurse specializing in IDD is responsible for assessing individual competence and is committed to the process of lifelong learning. Registered nurses specializing in IDD develop and maintain current knowledge and skills through formal and continuing education and seek available certification. APRNs specializing in IDD require specialized knowledge and skills obtained through formal and continuing education (i.e., Leadership Education in Neurodevelopmental Disabilities [LEND], meeting presentations on IDD health issues) related to the health care and management of conditions that are general or unique to the IDD population and their families.

All registered nurses are bound by a professional code of ethics (ANA, 2015b) and practice with highest respect and advocacy for the persons with IDD and families. The registered nurse is charged by the nurse practice act and empowered to promote the optimal life and environment for themselves and persons with IDD and their family. High-quality care will also be guided by research and evidence-based practice, in coordination through collaboration with the interdisciplinary team, family members, and consumers, to influence policy and practice. IDD registered nurses regulate themselves as individuals through a collegial process of peer review of practice. Peer evaluation fosters the refinement of knowledge, skills, and clinical decision-making at all levels and in IDD nursing practice. Self-regulation by the profession of nursing assures quality of performance, which is the heart of nursing's social contract (ANA, 2010a). IDD registered nurses recognize the larger scope of nursing's concern relative to the health of not only individuals and families, but also groups, communities, and IDD nurse roles as members of this nursing specialty. Registered nurses in IDD are fundamentally committed to respect for the individual, family, group, community, or population and their inherent dignity, worth, and uniqueness through advocating and protecting the rights, health, and safety of patients. The IDD registered nurse is accountable and responsible for decisions and actions that promote health and provide optimal patient care using such practices as shared decision making, self-determination, and interprofessional collaborations. Individually and collectively, the IDD registered nurse has the duty to maintain and promote *their own* health, safety, competence, personal and professional growth within an ethical work environment. The IDD registered nurse advances the profession beyond individual patient care through scientific and scholarly inquiry, professional standards development, and generation of policy reflecting social justice principles in collaboration with other professionals and communities, with the goal to reduce health disparities and protect human rights. Federal rights and protections as exemplified in the ADA, IDEIA, and Section 504 of the Rehabilitation Act serve as guidance for IDD nurses.

Registered nurses specializing in IDD nursing and members of various professions exchange knowledge and ideas about how to deliver high-quality health care, resulting in overlaps and constantly changing professional practice boundaries. This interprofessional team collaboration involves recognition of the expertise of others within and outside one's profession and referral to those providers when appropriate. Such collaboration also involves some shared functions and a common focus on one overall mission. By necessity, IDD nursing's scope of practice has flexible boundaries.

Registered nurses specializing in IDD regularly evaluate safety, effectiveness, and cost in the planning and delivery of nursing care to individuals with IDD. Nurses recognize that resources are limited and unequally distributed and that the potential for improving access to care requires innovative approaches, such as treating individuals with IDD remotely. APRNs in IDD nursing are uniquely qualified to assess, diagnose, and treat individuals with IDD locally and remotely in accordance with state-approved regulations. As members of a profession, registered nurses work toward equitable distribution and availability of healthcare services to individuals with IDD throughout the nation and the world.

THE CODE OF ETHICS FOR NURSES

The *Code of Ethics for Nurses with Interpretive Statements* ("The Code"; ANA, 2015b) serves as the ethical framework in nursing regardless of practice setting or role and provides guidance for the future. The provisions explicate key ethical concepts and actions for all nurses in settings that care for the healthcare consumer with IDD. Detailed descriptive interpretive statements for each of the nine provisions of the Code are available at www.nursingworld.org/codeofethics.

The *Code of Ethics for Nurses with Interpretive Statements* arises from the long, distinguished, and enduring moral tradition of modern nursing in the United States. It is foundational to nursing theory, practice, and praxis in its expression of the values, virtues, and obligations that shape, guide, and inform nursing as a profession. It establishes the ethical standard for the profession and provides a guide for nurses to use in ethical analysis and decision-making (ANA, 2015b, p. vii). The Code also describes the ethical characteristics of the professional nurse:

> Individuals who become nurses, as well as the professional organizations that represent them, are expected not only to adhere to the values, moral norms, and ideals of the profession but also to embrace them as a part of what it means to be a nurse. The ethical tradition of nursing is self-reflective, enduring, and distinctive. A code of ethics for the nursing profession makes explicit the primary obligations, values, and ideals of the profession. It provides normative, applied moral guidance for nurses in terms of what they ought to do, be, and seek. The values and obligations in the *Code of Ethics for Nurses* apply to nurses in all roles, in all forms of practice, and in all settings. In fact, it informs every aspect of the nurse's life (ANA, 2015b, p. vii).

The IDD registered nurse uses the *Code of Ethics for Nurses with Interpretive Statements* (ANA, 2015b) and the ANA Position Statement on the *Nurse's Role in Providing Ethically and Developmentally Appropriate Care to People With Intellectual and Developmental Disabilities* (ANA, 2018) to guide practice. The IDD population-specific provisions are below.

The nurse caring for the healthcare consumer with IDD will:

Provision 1—Practice compassion and respect for the dignity and uniqueness of the healthcare consumer with IDD. IDD nurses demonstrate compassion and respect for consumers with IDD by actively listening to their concerns, addressing them, and advocating for their choices and preferences. IDD nurses are guided by engaged decision-making with consumers with IDD and their families or guardians. IDD nurses will support and advocate for their voices to be heard.

- Deliver care in a manner that preserves and protects the autonomy, dignity, rights, values, beliefs, and practices of the healthcare consumer with IDD and their family.

- Support the expression of sexuality of the healthcare consumer with IDD in a manner that is consistent with the healthcare consumer's gender expression, native culture, religious upbringing, family values, level of maturity, and offer counseling as appropriate.
- Facilitate the self-determined decisions of the healthcare consumer with IDD in all healthcare settings. The concept of "dignity of risk" means that the healthcare consumer with IDD should be empowered to make an informed decision that others might not have chosen. This reflects a shared balance in decision-making with the consumer, in which all the treatment options are presented and the benefits and risks of each discussed with respect for the consumer's self-determination.
- Advocate for life-sustaining treatment or refusal/withdrawal of life-sustaining treatment decisions by the healthcare consumer with IDD and the family.
- Provide palliative care for serious and terminal illness when appropriate and agreed upon by the healthcare consumer with IDD and family; or works with a palliative care agency to provide appropriate, individualized care to the healthcare consumer with IDD and family.
- Provide or arrange for effective and appropriate palliative care for healthcare consumers with IDD who undergo tests or treatments for illnesses, have chronic conditions, or are at the end of life.
- Provide support and resources for end-of-life care, grief, and bereavement when healthcare consumers with IDD experience loss.

Provision 2—Be committed to the healthcare consumer with IDD, their family, and their community. IDD nurses' commitment can be shown with thorough plans to support the strengths and needs of the healthcare consumer with IDD, as well as providing resources to support the consumer and their family. Although the relationship and dedication are strong, the IDD nurse maintains a professional relationship with the healthcare consumer with IDD and family.

- Recognize the centrality of the healthcare consumer with IDD and family or legal guardians as core members of the healthcare team.
- Identify a surrogate for healthcare decisions in lieu of a formal guardianship process, when appropriate, and in accordance with local or state statutes.
- Advance the transitional care of the healthcare consumer with IDD and their family throughout the life course in health care and the community.

Provision 3—Protect, promote, and advocate for the rights, health, and safety of the healthcare consumer with IDD and their family. The nurse caring for the healthcare consumer with IDD maintains confidentiality and privacy unless reporting abuse or neglect as required by law. The IDD nurse will only disclose information pertinent to the care and well-being of the healthcare consumer with IDD with members of the team. The IDD nurse will ensure the healthcare consumer with IDD or their surrogate are aware of their rights and laws in accordance with ADA.

- Serve as an advocate for the healthcare consumer with IDD and family or legal guardians by developing their collective self-advocacy skills in areas of health and safety, for example, teaching the individual with IDD and family how to safely access transportation services that will facilitate their independence.
- Advocate for the healthcare consumer with IDD in self-determination decisions and engage the surrogate decision-maker for full discernment.
- Assist in assuring that the living arrangement for the healthcare consumer with IDD is the most appropriate and the least restrictive environment (LRE) possible.
- Assess the safety of the living conditions and arrangement and assist the consumer with IDD, family members, and caregivers on assessing for safety.

Provision 4—Be accountable and responsible to the nurse practice act, with decisions and actions to promote health and provide optimal care for the healthcare consumer with IDD and their family. The IDD nurse caring for a healthcare consumer with IDD may manage their care and relay information to the advanced practitioner or physician. If orders are placed, the nurse will verify that the treatment plan is appropriate for the healthcare consumer with IDD. If nursing tasks are delegated, the IDD nurse will confirm that the tasks are within the delegated person's scope of practice. For example, conducting a head to toe assessment would be inappropriate for nonlicensed personnel.

- Maintain a therapeutic and professional relationship with the healthcare consumer with IDD and their family that promotes appropriate professional role boundaries.
- Advocate for the decisions and actions that promote optimal care of the individual with IDD and family or legal guardians and, when appropriate, initiate referral to an organizationally recognized advocate.
- Assist in the referral process for local, state, regional, and federal assistance services and programs.

Provision 5—Promote health and safety for the IDD nurse; maintain competencies, as well as personal and professional development. Professional growth may be supported with certification in the IDD specialty or graduate level education in nursing with specialization in IDD nursing. Membership in IDD nursing organizations and interest groups is another professional venue for professional development. Seeking colleagues who specialize in IDD nursing as mentors is another professional growth option.

- Demonstrate a commitment to maintaining IDD nursing competencies and professional development while practicing personal self-care, sustaining healthy interpersonal relationships, and using stress-reduction methods and skills.
- Educate colleagues outside of the IDD specialty who provide health care to consumers with IDD and their families.

Provision 6—Work collaboratively to provide an ethical, safe, and high-quality work environment for him/herself and for the healthcare consumer with IDD and their family. Nurses will encourage a supportive work environment for themselves and settings for the healthcare consumer with IDD that is free from incivility. The work environment will allow for "safe spaces" to openly discuss concerns as identified in the *Healthy Nurse, Healthy Nation Initiative, Code of Ethics for Nurses with Interpretive Statements,* and *Nurse's Role in Providing Ethically and Developmentally Appropriate Care to People With Intellectual and Developmental Disabilities* (ANA, 2013d, 2015).

- Uphold confidentiality of the healthcare consumer with IDD and families within legal and regulatory parameters.
- Take appropriate action regarding instances of illegal, unethical, or incompetent behavior that can endanger or jeopardize the best interests of the healthcare consumer with IDD and their family.
- Work to prevent abuse or exploitation of the healthcare consumer with IDD and promptly respond to suspicion or evidence by reporting to appropriate authorities.
- Contribute to an environment that protects the healthcare consumer with IDD from sexual exploitation in the home, school, work, and community.

Provision 7—Advance the profession through scholarly inquiry, standards development, and influencing policy. The IDD nurse may pursue graduate-level education or certifications specific to IDD. IDD nurses are involved with conducting quality improvement or research projects to improve the quality of care and outcomes for the healthcare consumer with IDD and their family. IDD nurses participate in influencing policy-making or legislation for consumers with IDD and their families by contacting their state or local representatives to support initiatives that will benefit this vulnerable group.

- Question healthcare practices and institutional policies that are not in alignment with the optimal safety of the individual with IDD and family to promote organizational quality improvements using improvement science or systematic research.

- Contribute to the educational and vocational program recommendations and advocate for LRE to maximize the potential of the healthcare consumer with IDD.
- Serve as an advocate to ensure that the healthcare consumer with IDD receives coordinated, continuous, and accessible health care that is provided by a professional who is competent in managing the health concerns of healthcare consumers with IDD.

Provision 8—Work as a team with other providers to protect the rights, promote the health, and reduce disparities of the healthcare consumer with IDD and their family. The IDD nurse works with interdisciplinary teams to safeguard the rights of healthcare consumers with IDD to an LRE and to promote one's strengths, in accordance with the Every Student Succeeds Act, Section 504 of the Rehabilitation Act of 1973, ADA of 1990, and the state-level legislation such as California's Lanterman Developmental Disabilities Services Act (1969). IDD nurses advocate for programs and services that support the quality of life for individuals with IDD and their families.

- Participate in interdisciplinary teams to address ethical risks, benefits, and outcomes.
- Inform administrators or leaders of the risks, benefits, and outcomes of programs and decisions that affect equitable healthcare delivery to the healthcare consumer with IDD and their family.
- Contribute to the life course plan and advocate for the most appropriate employment or volunteer situation for the healthcare consumer with IDD. The nurse assists in identifying reasonable accommodations to maximize the healthcare consumer's performance and satisfaction with chosen employment or volunteer activity.

Provision 9—Will work with professional organizations to communicate values and incorporate social justice. IDD nurses who are members of DDNA or AAIDD are involved in promoting policies and legislation that improve access to care, provide for freedom of mobility, and decrease discrimination. IDD nurses who are members of other nursing professional organizations have opportunities to advocate for policies and initiatives that benefit and address the needs of individuals with IDD and their families.

- Respect the right of the healthcare consumer with IDD to self-determination by engaging them and their family in shared decision-making, unless the healthcare consumer's incapacity to participate in a specific decision is demonstrated and a surrogate decision-maker is legally required.
- Advocate for equitable health care for consumers with IDD and families in organizations and the community.
- Contribute to resolving ethical issues involving the healthcare consumer with IDD, colleagues, community groups, systems, and other stakeholders as evidenced by activities such as participating on ethics committees and influencing policymakers.

PROFESSIONAL REGISTERED NURSES TODAY: THE WHO OF IDD NURSING

Statistical Snapshot

The number of nurses identifying themselves as IDD nurses is unknown. The only national certification program for registered nurses specifically addressing individuals with IDD is through the DDNA, which claims about 1,300 members, including LPNs, associate-degree registered nurses, baccalaureate-prepared registered nurses, as well as APRNs and doctorally prepared nurses. Interdisciplinary organizations such as the AAIDD, American Academy for Cerebral Palsy and Developmental Medicine, and the International Association for the Scientific Study of Intellectual Disability count nurses among their membership. Additionally of interest is that the NASN Special Needs School Nurses Special Interest Group numbering 3,260 registered nurse members (NASN, 2019b). Those school nurses are not necessarily certified as IDD registered nurses, but it is an indication of the large number of school nurses who want to keep up with education and issues related to students with IDD. The Special Needs School Nurses Special Interest Group has a discussion list-serve that facilitates communication among members.

LICENSURE AND EDUCATION OF IDD REGISTERED NURSES

The IDD registered nurse is licensed and authorized by a state, commonwealth, or territory to practice nursing. IDD registered nurses, like all registered nurses, can take several pre-licensure educational routes. These educational options include nursing diploma, associate, and baccalaureate degrees. Entry-level registered nurses are prepared as generalists and often specialize following graduation and licensure. Continuing education programs and progressive work experience with individuals who have IDD enhance the IDD nurse's knowledge, skills, and abilities.

At the graduate level, few nursing education programs across the country offer specialization in IDD, and these programs are funded by the Maternal and Child Health Bureau, Department of Health and Human Services and are known as the Leadership Education in Neurodevelopmental and Related Disabilities (LEND). Many LEND programs are located in the University Centers of Excellence in Developmental Disabilities Education, Research and Service (UCEDD). A listing of these programs can be found on the Maternal and Child Health Bureau web site (mchb.hrsa.gov/training/ and click on Programs and Initiatives; from the home page, indicate "nursing" in the field asking for discipline).

IDD registered nurses with a Master's degree may continue their education toward the Doctor of Philosophy (PhD) degree or the Doctor of Nursing Practice (DNP) degree. The PhD graduate focuses on research and theory generation, as well as academic education. The DNP graduate focuses on clinical practice, quality assurance, and clinical outcome evaluation, as well as clinical education in academic and other settings.

There are many opportunities for nurses with graduate-level degrees who specialize in IDD nursing to engage in program development, consultation, policymaking, education, and research efforts. Nurses with an advanced degree specializing in IDD can be involved in leadership efforts to develop and implement nurse-led programs such as in early intervention, transition, and aging. Nurses with advanced degrees can be involved in policymaking and service system organizations at the state and federal levels that have wide-ranging and far-reaching effects that improve and expand services and programs available for individuals with IDD and their families. APRNs can provide consultation to interdisciplinary colleagues who work in practice settings such as medical centers and rehabilitation facilities on care issues involving individuals with IDD. APRNs may be asked to assist with the development of education programs and outreach training for staff on selected topics such as aggressive and challenging behaviors of individuals with IDD.

IDD APRNs, as nurse practitioners and clinical nurse specialists, can be members of interdisciplinary teams that provide direct services and coordination of care in specialty clinics associated with pediatric and adult-oriented medical centers. IDD nurses provide direct care and service coordination in programs that serve children with known or suspected developmental conditions and adults with IDD, such as autism spectrum disorder, brain injury, cerebral palsy, inborn errors of metabolism, seizure disorders, and many other pediatric neurological and genetic conditions.

Nurses who have advanced training in education can seek faculty and consultation positions within academic programs, such as the LEND training programs. Nursing administrative positions are available in community settings that serve individuals with IDD and their families, such as rehabilitation centers or other agencies that provide long-term services.

In some states, APRNs practice under full scope of practice given the shortages of primary and specialty care physicians (Bauer & Bodenheimer, 2017; Kirch & Petelle, 2017; Xue et al., 2018). By 2030, there could be a shortage of more than 100,000 physicians with the specialty fields of practice with the IDD field most significantly affected (Kirch & Petelle, 2017). It is projected there will be greater numbers of NPs practicing in rural and health professional shortage areas, and working with those who are insured by Medicaid, particularly in states wherein there are full scope of practice regulations (Bauer & Bodenheimer, 2017). Since individuals with IDD are likely to be included among those who do not have access to primary physicians, APRNs may become primary caregivers to many of these individuals. This is another indication that IDD nursing specialty education is needed.

Efforts to address underserved areas and populations are underway that can positively affect access to care for individuals with IDD. In January 2018, the Enhanced Nursing Licensure Compact (eNLC) was implemented and has been adopted by 30 states. Although narrow in scope as it affects registered nurses and LPNs/LVNs only (APRNs not included), nurses with licensure in an eNLC state can migrate to other eNLC member states without having to take the licensing examination of that state (National Council of State Boards of Nursing [NCSBN], 2018). The aim is to redirect nursing resources to underserved areas and for vulnerable populations wherein fluctuations in nursing resources exist. The eNLC is important for delivery of care, health-related education, and referrals, which can be done within the scope of practice for registered nurses and APRNs.

DEFINITIONS AND CONCEPTS RELATED TO COMPETENCE IN IDD NURSING

Competence in IDD nursing is based upon the standards of nursing practice generated by ANA, state boards of registered nursing, and specialty organizations. The ANA Professional Role Competence Position Statement (2014b) defines competence as "…performing successfully at an expected level and with "…an expected level of performance that integrates knowledge, skills, abilities, and judgment" (p. 3). In the ANA *Code of Ethics for Nurses with Interpretive Statements* (2015b), Provision 5.5 directly addresses the issue of competence and continuation of professional growth. Competence is referred to as "…a self-regarding duty" (p. 22). That is, nurses have a responsibility to "…maintain competence and strive for excellence in their nursing practice, whatever the role or setting" (p. 22).

The National Council of State Boards of Nursing defined competence as "the application of knowledge and the interpersonal, decision-making, and psychomotor skills expected for the practice role, within the context of public health" (NCSBN, 2005, p. 81). Competence is referred to as "a measure of performance that is the active, behavioral expression of expertise lying on a continuum from novice to expert (Bathisha, Wilson, & Potempa, 2018). Competence is composed of varied attributes, including judgment, critical thinking skills, and physical/behavioral skills. Competence is job related, situation related, and represents qualities that yield effective performance on the job.

Attributes associated with nurse competence, including IDD nursing competence, are the ability to integrate knowledge into practice, caring attitude, communication skills, critical thinking, professional experience, motivation, organizational environment, professionalism, and skills proficiency (Smith, 2012). Benner (1984) proposed a developmental model of competence, with stages from novice to expert, which posits that competence is also dependent on length of experience. More recently, deliberate practice, defined as activities undertaken "...aimed at improving one's competence and leading to expertise," is linked to competence (Bathish et al., 2018, p. 106).

Lifelong learning serves as the basis of deliberate practice and essential for achieving and maintaining competence. Because nursing education generally lacks content and experience in care of individuals with IDD, nurses must continually seek learning opportunities on the job through advanced educational preparation or combined with continuing education.

A variety of intrinsic and extrinsic factors influence competence in actual day-to-day nursing practice including IDD nursing practice. Quality care results from competence. Environmental factors may be supportive of competence or present challenges. For example, performing an assessment and physical examination on a cooperative patient may be a basic skill, but performing those activities with an individual with autism, a sensory disorder, and a communication disorder may necessitate a different set of knowledge, skills, and expertise.

There is little empirical data to inform care of individuals with IDD and to guide competence in nursing practice with this population.

However, evidence for practice can be sought by accessing the interdisciplinary literature and serving as a member of interdisciplinary teams. The majority of nurses entering into practice have little or no experience with children or adults with IDD, and many believe they will never encounter these persons in practice. However, as more individuals with IDD leave institutions and live in the community, nurses in all settings, including school nurses, will find themselves involved in providing services for the IDD population.

The registered nurse who specializes in IDD systematically enhances the quality and effectiveness of nursing practice by performing care according to quality standards and by meeting both generalist and specialist nursing competencies. These examples include the scope and standards of nursing practice published by ANA, such as gerontological nursing, pediatric nursing, psychiatric/mental health, public health nursing, genetics/genomic nursing, and school nursing practice. Other nursing subspecialty resources such as *Health Care Quality and Outcomes Guidelines for Nursing of Children, Adolescents, and Families* that denote excellence in pediatric nursing practice can be accessed for IDD nursing practice (Betz et al., 2018). Lifelong learning is a commitment to quality, requiring nurses to constantly reappraise their own practice and seek to upgrade knowledge and skills.

Evaluating Competence

Competence in nursing practice, including IDD nursing practice, must be evaluated by the individual nurse (self-assessment), nurse peers, and nurses in the roles of supervisor, coach, mentor, or preceptor. In addition, other aspects of nursing performance may be evaluated by professional colleagues and patients. Competence can be evaluated by using tools that capture objective and subjective data about the individual's knowledge base and actual performance and are appropriate for the specific situation and the desired outcome of the competence evaluation. However, no single evaluation tool or method can guarantee competence (ANA, 2014b).

Bachelor's and associate-level programs prepare nurses to meet general nursing competencies and to pass the NCLEX-RN licensing exams upon graduation (Kronk, Colbert, Smeltzer, & Blunt, 2019). Graduation from an accredited program and successful completion of the licensing exam represent to the public, consumers, and employers that the registered nurse is capable of general, competent, and safe nursing care. The IOM (IOM, 2011) recommends that all graduating registered nurses complete a nurse internship before entering into independent practice. Currently, this occurs mostly in the hospital setting, but nurse internships in community agencies serving individuals with IDD are needed. They would allow novice registered nurses to hone the basic skills they developed in training and apply them to the needs of the IDD population.

Continuing education and monitoring numbers of continuing education units have traditionally been the primary method for evaluating competence for practicing registered nurses, as well as many APRNs. As noted previously, nursing organizations such as the Developmental Disabilities Nurses Association (DDNA) offer certification of registered nurses (separate from APRN certification) as one method of evaluating competence of professional nurses working in specialized settings. Certification in IDD nursing can be found on the DDNA website (ddna.org/certification/).

IDD registered nurses evaluate their own nursing practice in relation to professional practice standards and evidence-based guidelines, and relevant statutes, rules, and regulations, identifying strengths and areas in need of further development. As part of the self-evaluation of practice, the registered nurse solicits feedback from healthcare consumers, family members or legal guardians, colleagues, and others, including direct care support professionals. Use of practice portfolios places the responsibility of maintaining competence on the individual nurse and can document experience in subspecialties (such as care of individuals with IDD), involvement in quality assurance efforts, and participation in professional interdisciplinary and nursing specialty organizations, as well as competencies not evaluated by other methods. The IDD nurse must also evaluate nursing care delegated to other professionals, direct care support professionals, unlicensed assistive personnel, or the family or legal guardians and document the effect of delegation on health outcomes.

Professional Trends and Issues

Nurses practicing in the field of IDD continue to refine and improve their care through clinical practice and advocacy. As practice in this field continues to evolve and advance, several areas will remain essential to provision of quality care to this vulnerable population, including cultural sensitivity, early assessment and identification, inclusion in schools and community, chronic illness, transition from pediatric to adult healthcare services, self-advocacy and self-determination, accessing and securing an equitable share of healthcare services, community living including environmental barriers, and genomics.

The most significant societal shift that has emerged in the past several decades has been the increase in cultural diversity of the nation's population (ANA, 2015a; Campinha-Bacote, 2011a,b; Leininger & McFarland, 2002; McFarland & Wehbe-Alamah, 2015). This pattern of diversity is also observed in the IDD population (Butler et al., 2016). This trend demands increased efforts by nurses to expand their cultural competence in adapting care to cultural norms that foster communication and positive health outcomes for this population, their families, and legal guardians.

Nurses also play a key role in the healthcare management of individuals with IDD throughout their lifetime. Technological medical advances have resulted in increased longevity for this population, resulting in a crucial need for nursing care that facilitates a smooth transition from pediatric to adult-oriented primary and specialty health services for individuals with IDD (Betz et al., 2015). In schools, for example, ITPs are started by age 16 for students who have IEPs, to plan their transition from school to community. ITPs are developed by multidisciplinary teams, which include school nurses when there are health-related issues, for example, bipolar disorder, diabetes, or seizure disorder. School nurses also can help students, and their guardians, with students' transition from pediatric to adult healthcare providers. The shift to adulthood also requires individualized counseling and coaching strategies to develop key self-advocacy skills that ensure their healthcare needs are met. Advocacy efforts also guide and support efforts that include individuals with IDD in making, to the extent possible, decisions regarding their health and well-being, including their goals for care at the end of life. More evidence is needed that focuses on effective assessment and intervention techniques for the unique needs of older persons with IDD, and particularly with those who develop dementia as a secondary diagnosis (Jaques et al., 2018).

The continued aging of the IDD population requires IDD nurses to prioritize care that is illness focused to health promotion and disease prevention. Specific nursing roles include creating environments conducive to health, involving stakeholders in planning health goals, and promoting self-care. New discoveries in genetic and genomic health care continue to demand that IDD nurses have essential competencies in this specialized clinical area. These IDD competencies will promote appropriate utilization of genetic care resources for innovative diagnostic procedures, genetic evaluation, counseling or risk assessment, and personalized, targeted drug and therapeutic interventions that might be indicated for the person with IDD and family.

New advances in information technology (IT) have the potential to provide expanded professional IDD nursing services to persons with IDD. Telehealth services can connect IDD nurses with individuals with IDD and their families in underserved and rural areas with a range of healthcare services and resources. Telehealth services may also benefit persons with IDD whose mobility impairments or fragile health status impede safe and accessible transportation to other healthcare facilities.

There is also an ongoing nursing shortage in the specialty of IDD nursing. Efforts are being made by public and private institutions to increase salaries for IDD registered nurses. Although IDD nurses' expert knowledge and skills are necessary to meet the unique healthcare needs of the IDD population, their compensation is less than that of nurses in other specialty areas (Augury, 2018). The basis for this discrepancy is unclear but may be related to "lack of recognition regarding this nursing specialty within the profession, ambiguous nature of the IDD nursing role, and significant gaps in research that clearly guide practice in this field" (Aubury, 2018, p. 26). Integration of IDD content into nursing curriculums will provide opportunities for novice nurses to discover the benefits and contributions that a career in caring for this population can provide to individuals with IDD, families, and society. Other opportunities for learning include membership in national professional organizations with subspecialty interest groups in IDD nursing. These are listed in Table 1.

TABLE 1 APRN Special Interest Groups for IDD

Advanced Practice Clinician (APC) Section of the Society for Developmental and Behavioral Pediatrics (SDBP)	The Advanced Practice Clinician Section of SDBP promotes the professional development of Advanced Practice Registered Nurses (APRN) working in Developmental and Behavioral Pediatrics.
NAPNAP SIG Developmental, Behavioral, and Mental Health (DBMH)	This SIG would be of interest for new and established APRNs in the field of IDD nursing. The NAPNAP DBMH SIG developed, vetted, and updated a comprehensive online resource library that is available for free and provides valuable information for IDD nurses: **dbmhresource.org**.
SDBP Nurse Practitioner SIG and NAPNAP DBMH SIG	The SDBP APC Section and the NAPNAP DBMH SIG have partnered to provide conference workshops and online learning modules for healthcare providers who work with children and adolescents with IDD and related disorders. The link below is available to all and a resource for nurses interested in IDD nursing: dbmhresource.org. The DBMH site management team is also available for contact at mentalhealth@napnap.org.

CREATING A SUSTAINABLE NURSING WORKFORCE

Scant data are available on the number of IDD nurses and projected numbers of IDD nurses needed to meet the ongoing and future comprehensive healthcare needs of individuals with IDD. Several reasons have been offered as to the lack of available data, which includes lack of resources to conduct national surveys and the transformative changes resulting from the deinstitutionalization movement. Deinstitutionalization, begun decades ago, has altered the practice of nurses who specialize in IDD nursing as care is no longer provided in easily identifiable institutional settings (S. Diane Moore, personal communication, October 15, 2018; O'Reilly et al., 2018). As noted, "The specialized field of nursing has arguably been subjected to a greater amount of policy and professional delegitimization than any other specialty field of nursing" (O'Reilly et al., 2018, p. e12258).

Data on the projected trends with professional nursing and interprofessional practice, US population health needs, and changes in the delivery of health services will have significant impact on the healthcare needs of individuals with IDD. These predicted changes will alter the professional practice opportunities of IDD nurses to respond to them (Auerbach, Staiger, & Buerhaus, 2018; Bauer, & Bodenheimer, 2017; Xue et al., 2018). These challenges are not unique to the United States (Delahunty, 2017; Trollor et al., 2018). The projected trends include the aging United States population, including seniors with IDD, shortages of the medical and nursing workforce, and the reform and retooling of the healthcare delivery system of care so that more care will be provided in the community, home, and remotely (Buerhaus, Skinner, Auerback, & Staiger, 2017; Robert Wood Johnson Foundation, 2013). All these projected changes will impact the access and quality of care provided to individuals with IDD.

Projections of the nursing workforce will vary according to the region in the United States according to Current Population Survey and the American Community Survey data from 1979 to 2014. Nursing shortages are expected in New England (Maine, Massachusetts, New Hampshire, Rhode Island, Vermont), whereas the region of South Central (Arkansas, Louisiana, Oklahoma, Texas) are expected to have robust and ongoing growth workforce supply (Auerbach et al., 2018; Ying et al., 2018). The projected workforce supply in regions nationwide suggest that access to health services for individuals with IDD will be affected by geographic region in the United States, not only for those who live in rural areas and health professional shortage areas. For areas where projected IDD nursing shortages are anticipated to occur, additional efforts with job recruitment and establishment of additional nursing education programs that include IDD content and specialization will be needed (Auerbach et al., 2018).

The retirement of the generation of baby boomer nurses will shift generational focus to millennials, who will become the largest segment of the nursing workforce (Auerbach et al., 2017). The retirement of experienced nurses of the baby boomer generation of approximately one million nurses will result in the loss of the valuable workforce assets of acquired knowledge and skills needed for the provision of nursing care, estimated at 1.7 million years of experience (Buerhaus et al., 2017). This projected loss of expertise and experience will be felt for the care provided to individuals with IDD. This projected gap in the quality of care provided can result in adverse consequences for individuals with IDD associated with increases in the rates of hospitalizations and emergency room visits and higher rates of complications, secondary conditions, and comorbidities (Kleier, 2016; Buerhaus et al., 2017).

NURSING EDUCATION

IDD consumer healthcare needs and the care environment are more complex in the 21st century. IDD nurses have to make more critical decisions; be adept at using a variety of sophisticated, life-saving technology and information management systems; coordinate care among a variety of professional and community agencies; help healthcare consumers manage their IDD and chronic illnesses; lead change from within their organizations; and affect national policy that has implications for individuals with IDD and their parents or guardians. Consequently, nursing students need to develop a broader range of competencies in the areas of health policy and healthcare financing (including understanding health insurance benefits), community and public health, leadership, quality improvement, information management, and systems thinking and their application to the IDD population, parents or guardians, as well as become excellent IDD clinicians (IOM, 2011).

According to the IOM (2011), in order to meet this demand, nurses, including IDD nurses, should achieve higher levels of education.

Innovative ways for nursing students to achieve their degrees online, using virtual, simulated, and competency-based learning are needed. Schools of nursing must build their capacities to prepare more graduate-level students to assume roles in advanced practice, leadership, teaching, and research in the field of IDD (IOM, 2011).

Nursing as a profession continues to face dilemmas in entry into practice, recognition of the autonomy of advanced practice, maintenance of competence, complexity of multistate licensure, and the appropriate educational credentials for licensure and professional certification. These dilemmas are true for nurses who specialize in IDD nursing. Employers who provide opportunities for professional development and continuing education promote a positive practice environment in which nurses can maintain and enhance skills and competencies.

This is an exciting time of progress and evolution for interprofessional education, long acknowledged as the model of excellence for the provision of care to persons with IDD and their parents or legal guardians. According to the AACN (1995, para 1), "interdisciplinary education is when two or more disciplines collaborate in the learning process with the goal of fostering interprofessional interactions that enhance the practice of each discipline." Students from differing professions learn what each brings to the IDD healthcare team and how each needs to foster communication, collaboration, conflict resolution, and mutual respect before graduation and entry into practice (ANA, 2015a, pp. 48–49).

TECHNOLOGICAL ADVANCES

Technology can drive effectiveness and efficiency, provide convenience, extend care to populations with little access to transportation, and serve as a major influence on how nurses practice (Huston, 2013; OECD, 2013). Technology can promote ease of data transparency and retrieval when designed and implemented in a manner that supports nurses' work responsibilities and workflow. Work environments include conventional locations—hospitals, clinics, schools, and healthcare consumer homes—as well as virtual spaces such as online discussion groups, email, interactive video, and virtual interaction (Cipriano, 2009). Ideally, technology will eliminate redundancy and duplication of documentation; reduce errors; eliminate interruptions for missing supplies, equipment, and medications; and ease access to data, thereby allowing the nurse more time with the patient (Cipriano, 2009). Perhaps one of the most daunting challenges for nurses will be to retain the human element in practice. Other challenges include balancing cost with benefits, the daunting task of training the nursing workforce with a plan for sustainment, and assuring ethical use of technology (Huston, 2013).

The IDD nurse recognizes that these technologies are continuously emerging. While it is impossible to know them all, the IDD nurse should be aware of the proliferation and evolution of potential devices that serve to support patients with IDD and their families—some that have evidence to support use and some that may not be evidence-based. The IDD nurse's technological role will be to inform patients with IDD and families, encouraging them to be informed by evidence rather than by commercials and social media outlets. Healthcare information technology (HIT) is a mainstay in hospitals, clinics, communities, and homes. IDD nurses are in a strategic position to tailor how to best use HIT while balancing the human element in practice by actively participating in designing nursing workflow in and around HIT.

Assistive technology (AT) refers to tools, equipment, or products that can help people with IDD successfully complete activities at school, home, work, and in the community. This can be as simple as a magnifying glass to improve vision or as complex as a digital communication system. Staying abreast with these AT treatment options requires close collaboration with the rehabilitation professionals, including physiatrists, physical therapists, occupational therapists, speech and language pathologists, vocational counselors, and family members. Collaboration with these team members allows the IDD nurse to individualize AT that is appropriate for each individual with IDD and family. IDD nurses who are knowledgeable and proficient with the use of AT are better equipped to assist in designing solutions that promote independence in the individual with IDD.

A wide assortment of assistive technologies exists to assist individuals with IDD to be more mobile, such as wheelchairs, reverse walkers, crutches, and orthotic devices. Individuals with sensory impairments now have access to a wide variety of AT devices that enhance and support vision and hearing abilities. Environmental modifications include the use of grab bars in showers, enlarged doorways and passages and ramps, and modification of shelving and counters enabling residential access. Durable medical equipment includes transfer benches for bathing and toilet assist bars to facilitate independence with ADL. Software programs are available to assist individuals with cognitive problems such as memory and learning challenges (American Foundation for the Blind, n.d.; Center on Technology and Disability, 2018; U.S. Department of Health and Human Services, National Institutes of Health, & Eunice Kennedy Shriver National Institute of Child Health and Human Development, 2018a).

Rehabilitative technologies (RT) and techniques, also referred to as AT, are designed to aid individuals, including those with IDD, to restore or improve function following an injury or debilitating health condition. These disabling health challenges can occur at any time over the life course of an individual with IDD. These rehabilitation technologies include the use of robots and the use of virtual environments. Musculoskeletal modeling and simulations, and motion analysis are used for the purposes of diagnostic analysis of movement problems. Technologies used for the recovery of movement through stimulation of the brain are transcranial direct current stimulation and transcranial magnetic stimulation (U.S. Department of Health and Human Services, National Institutes of Health, & Eunice Kennedy Shriver National Institute of Child Health and Human Development, 2018b).

The use of current and future technologies raises competence issues for IDD registered nurses in terms of understanding their appropriateness for delivery of services for individuals with IDD. Questions arise in terms of the practice expectations for IDD registered nurses and how to remain clinically competent with developments in the field of assistive and RTs. These questions involve not only the scope of practice expectations for IDD registered nurses but also access to the educational options to be competent in this area of practice. Issues to consider include:

- Should AT and RT classes be offered in nursing curriculum across medical conditions as elective or required? Rationale: Nurses know it exists and need to be aware of its potentials.
- Should AT/RT, as a testing section, be required to receive certification from DDNA?
- What type of continuing AT/RT classes (CME) are offered to IDD nurse specialists?
- What type of collaboration is available with the Rehabilitation Department to address AT/RT?

POPULATION FOCUS

Redefining Health and Well-Being for the Millennial Generation

The generation designated as millennials is composed of individuals ages 22–37 years born between 1981 and 1996 (U.S. Census Bureau, 2017). In 2019, the number of millennials was projected to reach 73 million and outnumber the baby boomer generation (72 million) for the first time (Fry, 2018). Relevant generational changes have been noted with the millennials in contrast to previous generations, which have implications for the provision of health services in the future for the population of individuals with IDD.

The current generation, referred to as "digital natives," has been raised with exposure to and use of technology beginning early in their childhood. Technology is used by millennials, depending on their level of cognitive functioning, for entertainment and educational purposes, to access personal and health-related resources, and for social communication. Nearly all millennials (97 percent) report that they access the Internet, and 92 percent own smartphones (Frey, Igielnik, & Patten, 2018; Jiang, 2018). Additionally, access to technology is not relegated to higher income groups; a recent survey revealed that approximately two-thirds of low-income youth had a mobile phone, and nearly 40 percent had a smartphone. Well-known Internet social media used by millennials include Facebook, Twitter, Linkedin, and Instagram (Stephens & Gunther, 2016).

The use of technology for health teaching, health monitoring, and communication have an important role in the provision of services to individuals with IDD and their families. IDD nurse specialists will need to adapt and accommodate technology in the provision of services to remain current and in touch with the needs of the individuals with IDD and families served. It is also incumbent upon nurses to be informed about the sources of information parents and consumers access and respond with replies based upon the best evidence. Issues pertaining to the controversies pertaining to vaccination and autism are apt examples of access to erroneous information and misconceptions (American Academy of Pediatrics, 2013; Krishna, 2018).

Baby Boomers: Health and Chronic Illness

The average life course of a person in the United States with IDD extends into the 60s (Janicki, Dalton, Henderson, & Davidson, 1999). In a study of the life expectancy of Finnish adults with mild ID was comparable to the general population; the life expectancy of those with moderate, severe, and profound ID was less than the general population (Patja, Livanainen, Vesala, Oksanen, & Ruoppila, 2000). This creates a growing population of individuals with IDD with a new set of needs in which IDD nurses must integrate new care delivery knowledge and skills. Individuals with IDD have a higher risk of developing chronic health conditions at younger ages than other adults due to the confluence of biological factors related to syndromes and associated disabilities. With poor access to adequate health care, as well as lifestyle and environmental issues, the physical health of individuals with IDD may be compromised. Furthermore, people with IDD may need additional services and support as they reach middle and older ages. These new trajectories in the population of individuals with IDD point to the increased complexity of problems and the need for increased knowledge of providers and IDD nurses about how to deal with complex issues of chronic illness and disability in individuals with IDD (Acharya, Schindler, & Heller, 2016).

In addition to IDD health and nursing care needs, parenting takes on a new set of circumstances. Many parents are having children later in life, resulting in an increased age of parent caregivers of individuals with IDD (Prouty, Alba, & Lakin, 2008). Parents of adult children with IDD have special needs that are different from parents of young, growing children with IDD. Future planning becomes a large part of meeting the needs of their loved ones who are younger than they are, while at the same time considering their own age-related changes and needs. The information and support from the IDD healthcare team in general and IDD nurses who play a significant role in coordinating care, in particular, can increase a parent caregiver's ability to advocate for care, increase confidence in their parenting, and assist with navigating the complex array of services.

It is important for all nurses who work in the IDD communities to recognize the intergenerational differences and healthcare demands of aging parents along with their adult children with IDD. Just as aging people with IDD are likely to bring to their healthcare encounter a set of complex chronic illnesses that are associated with age, parent caregivers also experience increased challenges to physical functioning, health status, and level of stress (Anderson et al., 2018; Carling-Jenkins, Torr, Iacono, & Bigby, 2012; Chou, Chiao, & Fu, 2011). Families of children with IDD generally favor a lifetime assistance model—planning for the future and transfer of care (Hewitt et al., 2010). Families caring for an adult child with a disability can be viewed in context. A family-centered approach to integrating care, connecting aging parents with needed services for themselves and their child, can be best implemented by IDD nurses with advanced knowledge about disabilities, aging, chronic illness, and psychosocial needs of families. Family-Centered Care (FCC) is a philosophical and systematic approach to serving the family as a unit (Al-Motlaq et al., 2018), knowing that parent-caregivers and children are all stakeholders in meeting the needs of the individual with IDD.

A model that helps bring individuals with IDD, when able, and parents into the decision-making process is shared decision-making (SDM) (Charles, Gafni, & Whelan, 1997) and informed shared decision-making (ISDM) (Towle, Godolphin, Grams, & La Marre, 2006). Information sharing is a prerequisite to treatment decisions made by all stakeholders who have reached consensus. Interdisciplinary teams, including individuals with IDD and family members, need to work with both caregivers and their children with IDD to support healthcare decisions and self-care independence. In the event that the current living arrangement is no longer safe or optimum, decision-making for alternative placement with greater supervision and medical oversight is needed. IDD nurses with advanced practice skills are key to guide the ISDM process.

Parents approaching retirement age who have adult children with IDD who may also be baby boomers have spent a lifetime of caring for the health and welfare of their children with IDD. These families often first come to the attention of the aging network through referrals from hospital discharge planners, friends, and neighbors, especially when the older parents need support due to age-related changes in health and function. One of the challenges of the aging population of baby boomers with IDD is that throughout their lives, healthcare decisions have not always been their own. Today, members of the IDD team, including IDD nurses, are learning to include the individual with IDD as an equal partner and developing necessary skills to involve individuals with IDD as partners in care and decision-making (Moulton & King, 2010; Nickel, Weinberger, Guze, & Patient Partnership in Healthcare Committee of the American College of Physicians, 2018). IDD nurses play an integral role in understanding how best to support families and individuals with IDD in the shared decision-making process. These decision-making processes result in choices about health and health care with the support of family, healthcare professionals, and sometimes other stakeholders.

Adults aging with IDD are more likely than adults in the general population to have received lifelong services and supports. An estimated 71 percent of individuals with IDD live with their family caregivers; 24 percent have caregivers aged 60 years and older, while another 35 percent have caregivers aged 41–59 years. Only 13 percent of adults with IDD live in supervised residential settings (Braddock, Hemp, Tanis, Wu, & Haffer, 2017). In 2014, there were nearly 100,000 individuals with IDD on waiting lists for residential out-of-home services, and over 216,000 estimated to be waiting for any type of long-term services and supports (Larson et al., 2017).

Services for adults and aging adults with IDD have transformed over the past decades from segregated services; to individualized and person-centered planning for older adults that provide training in different activities in the communities and goal setting within their circle of support; to more emphasis on the rights to full inclusion in the community, universal design, and supported decision-making (Federal Register, 2014). These types of services are woefully in need of competent IDD nurses and an array of providers who are aware of the connection between aging and IDD.

As services in the United States evolve, the demand for nursing leadership in caring for individuals with IDD grows, and especially the need for IDD APRNs with the knowledge and skill that is required to meet the changing health needs of individuals with IDD and families. Increased supports for families are integral to helping the many adults with IDD who are living at home with family members. Challenges will occur as there is more pressure on community-based systems to supply a workforce that can support people aging with and into disability. There is a growing recognition of family-centered services, supportive decision-making, and interdependence between people across generations. Finally, a need exists for research on better ways to bridge aging and disability (Tripp, Whitehead, Crowe, Mirfin-Veitch, & Daffue, 2019).

SUMMARY OF THE SCOPE OF IDD NURSING PRACTICE

The dynamic nature of the healthcare practice environment and the growing body of nursing research provide both the impetus and the opportunity for IDD nursing to ensure competent nursing practice in all settings for all individuals with IDD and to promote ongoing professional development that enhances the quality of nursing practice. *Intellectual and Developmental Disabilities Nursing: Scope and Standards of Practice,*

3rd Edition, assists that process by delineating the professional scope and standards of practice and responsibilities of all professional registered nurses engaged in IDD nursing practice, regardless of setting. As such, it can serve as a basis for:

- Quality improvement systems;
- Regulatory systems;
- Healthcare reimbursement and financing methodologies;
- Development and evaluation of nursing service delivery systems and organizational structures
- Certification activities;
- Nursing education guidance;
- Research guidance;
- Position descriptions and performance appraisals;
- Agency policies, procedures, and protocols;
- Educational offerings; and
- Establishing the legal standard of care.

Standards of Professional Nursing Practice

SIGNIFICANCE OF STANDARDS

The Standards of Professional Nursing Practice are authoritative statements of the duties that all registered nurses, regardless of role, population, or specialty, are expected to perform competently. The standards published herein may be utilized as evidence of the standard of care, with the understanding that application of the standards is context dependent. The standards are subject to change with the dynamics of the nursing profession, as new patterns of professional practice are developed and accepted by the nursing profession and the public. In addition, specific conditions and clinical circumstances may also affect the application of the standards at a given time (e.g., during a natural disaster). The standards are subject to formal, periodic review and revision.

The competencies that accompany each standard may be evidence of compliance with the corresponding standard. The list of competencies is not exhaustive. Whether a particular standard or competency applies depends upon the circumstances. The competencies are presented for the registered nurse level and are applicable to *all* nurses who specialize in IDD. Standards may include additional competencies delineated for the graduate-level prepared registered nurse, a category that also includes APRNs. In some instances, additional discrete competencies applicable only to APRNs may be included. These standards apply to the nursing care of individuals with IDD of all ages, cultures, socioeconomic backgrounds, and medical diagnoses. They further apply to any health care, education, residential, or community setting where healthcare consumers with IDD might be. The competencies have been developed to represent quality practice and performance in the nursing care of healthcare consumers with IDD.

Standards of Practice for IDD Nurses

STANDARD 1. ASSESSMENT

The registered nurse who specializes in IDD collects comprehensive data pertinent to the healthcare consumer's health and the situation.

Competencies
The IDD registered nurse:

- Collects pertinent data, including but not limited to demographics, social determinants of health, health disparities, and physical, functional, psychosocial, emotional, cognitive, sexual, cultural, age-related, environmental, spiritual/transpersonal, and economic assessments in a systematic, ongoing process with compassion and respect for the inherent dignity, worth, and unique attributes of every person. This may involve observation, interviewing, and the use of screening and assessment tools. Diagnostic tests may be used as part of the assessment process if the nurse has specific training in that area (e.g., developmental diagnostic testing).
- Uses analytical models and problem-solving tools that are appropriate for healthcare consumers with IDD.
- Recognizes the importance of the assessment parameters identified by WHO (World Health Organization), *Healthy People 2030*, or other organizations that influence nursing practice, in particular those for conditions that result in an IDD.
- Integrates knowledge from global and environmental factors into the assessment process.
- Elicits the healthcare consumer with IDD's values, preferences, expressed and unexpressed needs, and knowledge of the healthcare situation along with that of their family or legal guardians.

- Involves the healthcare consumer with IDD, family or legal guardians, other healthcare and interdisciplinary professionals and paraprofessionals, and the work and home environment, as appropriate, in holistic data collection.
- Recognizes the impact of one's own personal attitudes, values, and beliefs on the assessment process.
- Identifies barriers to effective communication based on psychosocial, literacy, financial, and cultural considerations.
- Assesses the impact of family dynamics on the healthcare consumer with IDD's health and wellness.
- Engages the healthcare consumer with IDD, their family or legal guardians, and other interprofessional team members in holistic, culturally sensitive data collection.
- Prioritizes data collection based on the healthcare consumer with IDD's immediate condition or the anticipated needs of the healthcare consumer with IDD or situation.
- Uses evidence-based assessment techniques, instruments, tools, available data, information, and knowledge relevant to the situation to identify patterns and variances, including, but not limited to, genetic studies, special serum screening (e.g., cystic fibrosis, Tay–Sachs, sickle cell disease), nutritional needs and metabolic functioning, and any other condition-specific data measures.
- Synthesizes all data, information, and knowledge from the healthcare consumer with IDD, family members or legal guardians, the interprofessional team, and individual's environment that is relevant to the situation to identify patterns and variances. This may involve data and information from the school, work site, and residential setting.
- Applies ethical, legal, and privacy guidelines and policies to the collection, maintenance, use, and dissemination of data and information.
- Recognizes the healthcare consumers with IDD have authority over their own health by honoring their care preferences. As legally appropriate, a guardian may be involved in identifying and expressing those preferences.

- Documents relevant data accurately and in a manner accessible to the interprofessional team and family members.

ADDITIONAL COMPETENCIES FOR THE GRADUATE-LEVEL PREPARED REGISTERED NURSE WHO SPECIALIZES IN IDD

In addition to the registered nurse competencies, the graduate-level prepared registered nurse:

- Assesses the effect of interactions among individuals, family or legal guardians, community, and social systems on health and illness of the healthcare consumer with IDD.
- Synthesizes the results and information leading to clinical understanding.

ADDITIONAL COMPETENCIES FOR THE APRN WHO SPECIALIZES IN IDD

In addition to the competencies of the registered nurse and the graduate-level prepared registered nurse, the APRN who specializes in IDD:

- Initiates diagnostic tests and procedures relevant to the healthcare consumer with IDD's current status.
- Uses advanced assessment, knowledge, and skills to maintain, enhance, or improve health conditions for the healthcare consumer with IDD.

STANDARD 2. DIAGNOSIS

The registered nurse who specializes in IDD analyzes assessment data to determine diagnoses, problems, and issues.

Competencies

The IDD registered nurse:

- Identifies actual or potential risks to the healthcare consumer with IDD's health and safety or barriers to health, which may

include but are not limited to interpersonal, systematic, cultural, or environmental circumstances.
- Uses assessment data, standardized classification systems, technology, and clinical decision support tools to articulate actual or potential diagnoses, problems, and issues.
- Verifies the diagnoses, problems, and issues with the individual with IDD, family or legal guardians, community, population, and interprofessional colleagues.
- Prioritizes diagnoses, problems, and issues based on mutually established goals to meet the needs of the healthcare consumer with IDD across the health–illness continuum.
- Documents diagnoses, problems, and issues in a manner that facilitates the determination of the expected outcomes and plan.

ADDITIONAL COMPETENCIES FOR THE GRADUATE-LEVEL PREPARED REGISTERED NURSE WHO SPECIALIZES IN IDD

In addition to the competencies of the registered nurse, the graduate-level prepared registered nurse who specializes in IDD:

- Uses information and communication technologies to analyze diagnostic practice patterns of nurses and other members of the interprofessional healthcare team.
- Employs aggregate-level data to articulate diagnoses, problems, and issues of healthcare consumers with IDD and organizational systems.

ADDITIONAL COMPETENCIES FOR THE APRN WHO SPECIALIZES IN IDD

In addition to the competencies of the registered nurse and the graduate-level prepared registered nurse, the APRN who specializes in IDD:

- Formulates a differential diagnosis based on the assessment (including developmental), history, physical examination, and diagnostic test results.
- Systematically compares the health history, clinical findings, and variations in developmental events when formulating differential

diagnoses, interventions, and a plan of care that is cognizant of expected outcomes for a specific diagnosis (e.g., Down syndrome).
- Serves as a consultant to the registered nurse and other staff in developing and maintaining competence in the diagnostic process.
- Analyzes accessibility and availability of services, barriers to adequate health care, specific populations at high risk, health promotion needs for specific populations, and environmental hazards that may affect the health of healthcare consumers with IDD.

STANDARD 3. OUTCOMES IDENTIFICATION

The registered nurse who specializes in IDD identifies expected outcomes for a plan individualized to the healthcare consumer with IDD and the situation.

Competencies
The IDD registered nurse:

- Engages the healthcare consumer with IDD, family or legal guardians, interprofessional team, and others in partnership to identify expected outcomes.
- Formulates culturally sensitive expected outcomes derived from assessments and diagnoses.
- Uses clinical expertise and current evidence-based practice to identify health risks, benefits, costs, and expected trajectory of the condition.
- Engages in shared decision-making with the healthcare consumer with IDD and their family or legal guardians to define expected outcomes integrating the healthcare consumer with IDD and their family members or legal guardians' culture, values, and ethical considerations.
- Generates a time frame for the attainment of expected outcomes.
- Develops expected outcomes that facilitate coordination of care and person-centered care as appropriate.

- Modifies expected outcomes based on the evaluation of the status (i.e., health, social, living, economic, and legal) of the healthcare consumer with IDD and situation.
- Documents expected outcomes as measurable goals.
- Evaluates the actual outcomes in relation to expected outcomes, safety, and quality standards.

Additional Competencies for the Graduate-Level Prepared Registered Nurse Who Specializes in IDD, Including the APRN Who Specializes in IDD

In addition to the competencies of the registered nurse, the graduate-level prepared registered nurse or APRN who specializes in IDD:

- Defines expected outcomes that incorporate cost, clinical effectiveness, and legal and ethical boundaries among the individual with IDD, family or legal guardians, and healthcare providers, and are aligned with the outcomes identified by members of the interprofessional team.
- Differentiates outcomes that require care process interventions from those that require system-level actions.
- Integrates scientific evidence and best practices to achieve expected outcomes.
- Advocates for outcomes that reflect the healthcare consumer's culture, values, and ethical concerns.

STANDARD 4. PLANNING

The registered nurse who specializes in IDD develops a plan that prescribes strategies and alternatives to attain expected, measurable outcomes.

Competencies

The IDD registered nurse:

- Develops an individualized, holistic, evidence-based plan in partnership with the healthcare consumer with IDD, their family

or legal guardians, and interprofessional team considering the person's characteristics or situation, including but not limited to values, beliefs, spiritual and health practices, preferences, choices, chronological age and developmental level, coping style, culture, available technology, and the LRE.
- Establishes the plan priorities with the healthcare consumer with IDD, their family or legal guardians, and interprofessional team.
- Advocates for responsible and appropriate use of interventions to minimize unwarranted or unwanted treatment and healthcare consumer suffering.
- Prioritizes elements of the plan based on the assessment of the healthcare consumer with IDD's level of risk and safety needs.
- Includes evidence-based strategies in the plan to address each of the identified diagnoses, problems, or issues. These strategies may include but are not limited to:
  - Promotion and restoration of health,
  - Prevention of illness, injury, and disease,
  - Facilitation of healing,
  - Alleviation of suffering, and
  - Supportive care
- Incorporates an implementation pathway that describes steps and milestones.
- Identifies cost and economic implications of the plan on the healthcare consumer with IDD, family or legal guardians, caregivers, or other affected parties.
- Integrates current scientific evidence, trends, and research affecting comprehensive care of healthcare consumers of all ages with IDD into the planning process.
- Uses the plan to provide direction to family members or legal guardians and other members of the healthcare and interprofessional team.
- Develops a plan that reflects compliance with current statutes, rules and regulations, and standards affecting comprehensive care of healthcare consumers of all ages with IDD into the planning process.

- Investigates practice settings and safe space and time for the nurse and the healthcare consumer with IDD to explore suggested, potential, and alternative options.
- Modifies the plan according to the ongoing assessment of the healthcare consumer with IDD's response and other outcome indicators.
- Documents the plan using standardized, person-first language or recognized terminology.

Additional Competencies for the Graduate-Level Prepared Registered Nurse Who Specializes in IDD

In addition to the competencies of the registered nurse, the graduate-level prepared registered nurse who specializes in IDD:

- Designs strategies and tactics to meet the multifaceted and complex needs of healthcare consumers with IDD or others.
- Leads the design and development of interprofessional processes to address the identified diagnoses, problems, or issues.
- Designs innovative nursing practices.
- Participates actively in the development and continuous improvement of systems that support the planning process.

Additional Competencies for the APRN Who Specializes in IDD

In addition to the competencies of the registered nurse and graduate-level prepared registered nurse, the APRN who specializes in IDD:

- Integrates assessment strategies, screening and diagnostic strategies, and therapeutic interventions that reflect current evidence-based knowledge and practice.
- Selects or designs strategies to meet the multifaceted and complex needs of healthcare consumers with IDD.
- Includes in the plan a synthesis of the values and beliefs of the healthcare consumer with IDD regarding nursing, medical, social, and educational therapies.

- Leads the design and development of interprofessional processes to address the identified diagnosis, situation, or issue.
- Participates actively in the development and continuous improvement of organizational systems that support the planning process.
- Supports the integration of clinical, human, and financial resources to enhance and complete the decision-making and evaluation processes.
- Serves as a consultant to the registered nurse to plan development, priority setting, cost-benefit analysis, and identification of resources, as needed.
- Collaborates with the registered nurse and other members of the interprofessional team, including family team members, and in partnership with the community, derives community-focused plans that are based on identified problems, conditions, or needs that build on the strengths of the community.
- Develops plans that ensure continuity of care and minimize or eliminate gaps and duplications of services.

STANDARD 5. IMPLEMENTATION

The registered nurse who specializes in IDD implements the identified plan.

Competencies

The IDD registered nurse:

- Partners with the healthcare consumer with IDD, their family or legal guardians, significant others, and caregivers as appropriate to implement the plan in a safe, effective, efficient, timely, patient-centered, and equitable manner (IOM, 2010).
- Integrates interprofessional team partners in implementation of the plan through collaboration and communication across the continuum of care.
- Demonstrates caring behaviors to develop therapeutic relationships with healthcare consumers with IDD, significant others, and groups of people receiving care.

- Provides culturally congruent, holistic, and person-centered care that focuses on the healthcare consumer with IDD and addresses and advocates for the needs of diverse populations across the life course.
- Uses evidence-based interventions and strategies to achieve the mutually identified goals and outcomes specific to the problem or needs.
- Integrates critical thinking and technology solutions to implement the nursing process to collect, measure, record, retrieve, trend, and analyze data and information to enhance nursing practice and healthcare consumer outcomes.
- Uses community resources and systems to implement the plan.
- Collaborates with nursing colleagues and other healthcare providers from diverse backgrounds to implement and integrate the plan.
- Accommodates different styles of communication used by healthcare consumers with IDD, families or legal guardians, members of the interprofessional team, and other healthcare providers.
- Delegates according to the health, safety, and welfare of the healthcare consumer with IDD and considering the circumstance, person, task, direction or communication, supervision, evaluation, as well as the state nurse practice act regulations, institution, and regulatory entities while maintaining accountability for the care.
- Promotes the capacity of the healthcare consumer with IDD to achieve the optimal level of participation and problem-solving.
- Documents implementation and any modifications, including accommodations and changes or omissions, of the identified plan.

ADDITIONAL COMPETENCIES FOR THE GRADUATE-LEVEL PREPARED REGISTERED NURSE WHO SPECIALIZES IN IDD

In addition to the competencies of the registered nurse, the graduate-level prepared registered nurse who specializes in IDD:

- Uses systems, organizations, and community resources to lead effective changes and implement the plan.

- Applies quality principles while articulating methods, tools, performance measures, and standards as they relate to implementation of the plan.
- Translates evidence into practice.
- Leads interprofessional teams that include family team members to communicate, collaborate, and consult effectively.
- Demonstrates leadership skills that emphasize ethical and critical decision-making, effective working relationships, and systems perspective.
- Serves as a consultant to provide additional insight and potential solutions.
- Uses theory-driven approaches to effect organizational or system change.

Additional competencies for the APRN who specializes in IDD

In addition to the competencies of the registered nurse and graduate-level prepared nurse, the APRN who specializes in IDD:

- Uses prescriptive authority, procedures, referrals, treatments, and therapies in accordance with state and federal laws and regulations.
- Facilitates use of systems, organizations, and community resources to implement the plan.
- Uses advanced communication skills to promote relationships between nurses and healthcare consumers with IDD, to provide a context for open communication about the healthcare consumer's experiences, and to improve healthcare consumer outcomes.
- Participates actively in the development and continuous improvement of systems that support implementation of the plan.
- Prescribes traditional and integrative evidence-based treatments, therapies, and procedures that are compatible with the healthcare consumer with IDDs' cultural preferences and norms.
- Prescribes evidence-based pharmacological agents and treatments according to clinical indicators and results of screening, diagnostic, and laboratory tests.

- Supports collaboration with nursing colleagues and other members of the interprofessional team to implement the plan.
- Provides clinical consultation for healthcare consumers with IDD and professionals related to complex clinical cases to improve care and patient outcomes.
- Implements the plan using principles of project or systems management.

STANDARD 5A. COORDINATION OF CARE

The registered nurse who specializes in IDD coordinates care delivery. Coordination of care requires that the nurse work closely with individuals with IDD, families, community resources, and other health systems.

Competencies
The IDD registered nurse:

- Organizes the components of the plan.
- Engages in shared decision-making with the consumer with IDD and the family or legal guardians, as appropriate, to help manage health care based on mutually agreed-upon outcomes.
- Manages a healthcare consumer with IDD's care in order to reach mutually agreed-upon outcomes.
- Engages healthcare consumers with IDD in self-care to achieve preferred goals for quality of life in partnership with family or legal guardians.
- Assists the healthcare consumer with IDD and the family or legal guardians, as appropriate, to identity options for care.
- Communicates with the healthcare consumer with IDD, family or legal guardians, interprofessional team, and community-based personnel to effect safe transitions in continuity of care.
- Advocates for the delivery of dignified and holistic care by the interprofessional team that includes family team members.
- Documents the coordination of care.
- Makes referrals to other disciplines as needed.

- Provides direction or supervision to ancillary and unlicensed personnel who provide health care to healthcare consumers with IDD and their families or legal guardians.
- Keeps the healthcare consumer with IDD and family or legal guardian (and direct care support professionals when present) informed about the health status of the consumer.
- Keeps the healthcare consumer with IDD and the family or legal guardians informed about healthcare resources that are available.
- Employs strategies to promote health in home and community settings that are safe and utilize the least restrictive alternatives.

ADDITIONAL COMPETENCIES FOR THE GRADUATE-LEVEL PREPARED REGISTERED NURSE WHO SPECIALIZES IN IDD

In addition to the competencies of the registered nurse, the graduate-level prepared registered nurse who specializes in IDD:

- Provides leadership in the coordination of interprofessional health care for integrated delivery of healthcare consumer services to achieve safe, effective, efficient, timely, patient-centered, and equitable care (IOM, 2010).

ADDITIONAL COMPETENCIES FOR THE APRN WHO SPECIALIZES IN IDD

In addition to the competencies of the registered nurse and graduate-level prepared registered nurse, the APRN who specializes in IDD:

- Manages identified consumer panels or populations.
- Serves as the healthcare consumer with IDD's primary care provider and coordinator of healthcare services in accordance with the state and federal laws and regulations.
- Provides leadership in the coordination of interprofessional health care for integrated delivery of healthcare services for the healthcare consumer with IDD.
- Synthesizes data and information to prescribe and provide necessary system and community support measures, including modifications of environments.
- Coordinates system and community resources that enhance delivery of care across continuums.

STANDARD 5B. HEALTH TEACHING AND HEALTH PROMOTION

The registered nurse who specializes in IDD employs strategies to promote health, prevention of secondary disability, and a safe environment.

Competencies
The IDD registered nurse:

- Provides opportunities for the healthcare consumer with IDD to identify needed healthcare promotion, disease prevention, and self-management topics.
- Provides health teaching that addresses such topics as healthy lifestyles, risk-reducing behaviors, developmental needs, ADL, self-care concepts, and preventive self-care.
- Uses health promotion and health teaching methods in collaboration with the healthcare consumer with IDD's values, beliefs, health practices, developmental level, learning needs, readiness and ability to learn, language preference, spirituality, culture, and socioeconomic status.
- Uses feedback and evaluations from the healthcare consumer with IDD, family or legal guardians, and caregivers, as appropriate, to determine the effectiveness of the employed strategies.
- Uses technologies to communicate health promotion and disease prevention information to the healthcare consumer with IDD and their families or legal guardians in a variety of settings.
- Provides healthcare consumers with IDD and their families or legal guardians with information about intended effects and potential adverse effects of the plan of care.
- Engages consumer alliance and advocacy groups in health teaching and health promotion activities for healthcare consumers with IDD.
- Provides anticipatory guidance to healthcare consumers with IDD and their families or legal guardians to promote health and prevent or reduce the risk of negative health outcomes.

ADDITIONAL COMPETENCIES FOR THE GRADUATE-LEVEL PREPARED REGISTERED NURSE, INCLUDING THE APRN WHO SPECIALIZES IN IDD

In addition to the competencies of the registered nurse, the graduate-level prepared registered nurse or APRN who specializes in IDD:

- Synthesizes empirical evidence on risk behaviors, gender roles, learning theories, behavioral change theories, motivational theories, translational theories for evidence-based practice, epidemiology, and other related theories and frameworks when designing health education information and programs.
- Evaluates health information resources for applicability, accuracy, readability, and comprehensibility to help healthcare consumers with IDD, family or legal guardians, and other members of the interprofessional team access quality health information.
- Conducts personalized health teaching and counseling considering comparative effectiveness research recommendations.
- Designs health information and healthcare consumer education appropriate to the developmental level, learning needs, readiness to learn, and cultural values and beliefs of the healthcare consumer with IDD.
- Provides anticipatory guidance to individuals with IDD, families or legal guardians, groups, and communities to promote health and prevent or reduce the risk of health problems.

STANDARD 6. EVALUATION

The registered nurse who specializes in IDD evaluates progress toward attainment of goals and outcomes.

Competencies

The IDD registered nurse:

- Conducts a holistic, systematic, ongoing, and criterion-based evaluation of the goals and outcomes in relation to the structure, processes, and timeline prescribed in the plan.

- Collaborates with the healthcare consumer with IDD, family or legal guardians, members of the interprofessional team, and others involved in the care or situation in the evaluation process.
- Determines, in partnership with the healthcare consumer with IDD and other stakeholders, the patient-centeredness, effectiveness, efficiency, safety, timeliness, and equitability (IOM, 2001) of the strategies in relation to the responses to the plan and attainment of outcomes. Other defined criteria (e.g., Quality and Safety Education for Nurses) may be used as well.
- Uses ongoing assessment data to revise the diagnosis, outcomes, plans, and implementation strategies.
- Shares evaluation data and conclusions with the healthcare consumer with IDD and other stakeholders in accordance with federal and state regulations.
- Participates in assessing and assuring the responsible and appropriate use of interventions in order to minimize unwarranted and unwanted treatment and healthcare consumer suffering.
- Documents the results of the evaluation.

ADDITIONAL COMPETENCIES FOR THE GRADUATE-LEVEL PREPARED REGISTERED NURSE, INCLUDING THE APRN WHO SPECIALIZES IN IDD

In addition to the competencies of the registered nurse, the graduate-level prepared registered nurse or the APRN who specializes in IDD:

- Evaluates the accuracy of the diagnosis and the effectiveness of the interventions and other variables in relation to the attainment of expected outcomes.
- Synthesizes evaluation data from the healthcare consumer with IDD, their family or legal guardians, caregivers, community, population, and institution to determine the effectiveness of the plan.
- Engages in a systematic evaluation process to revise the plan to enhance its effectiveness.
- Uses results of the evaluation to make or recommend process, policy, procedure, or protocol revisions when warranted.

Standards of Professional Performance for IDD Nurses

STANDARD 7. ETHICS

The registered nurse who specializes in IDD practices ethically.

Competencies
The IDD registered nurse:

- Uses the *Code of Ethics for Nurses with Interpretive Statements* (ANA, 2015b) to guide practice.
- Practices compassion and respect for the inherent dignity, worth, and unique attributes of the healthcare consumer with IDD and family or legal guardians.
- Is committed to the healthcare consumer with IDD, their family or legal guardians, circle of support, community, or populations.
- Recognizes the centrality of the healthcare consumer with IDD and family or legal guardians as core members of any healthcare team.
- Upholds confidentiality of the healthcare consumer with IDD within legal and regulatory parameters.
- Serves as advocate for the healthcare consumer with IDD and family or legal guardians by supporting the development of their advocacy and self-advocacy skills.
- Maintains a therapeutic and professional relationship with the healthcare consumer with IDD within appropriate professional role boundaries.

- Protects, promotes, and advocates for the health and safety of the healthcare consumer with IDD and their family or legal guardians.
- Has authority, accountability, and responsibility for the nurse practice act; makes decisions; and takes actions consistent with the obligation to promote health and provide optimal care of the healthcare consumer with IDD and their family or legal guardians.
- Owes the same duties to self as to others, including the responsibility to promote health and safety for consumers with IDD and their family or legal guardians, preserve wholeness of character and integrity, maintain competence, and continue personal and professional growth.
- Establishes, maintains, and improves the ethical environment of the work setting and conditions of employment or volunteer activities that are conducive to safe, quality health care for the consumer with IDD, family or legal guardians, and colleagues.
- Takes appropriate action regarding instances of illegal, unethical, or inappropriate behavior that can endanger or jeopardize the best interests of the healthcare consumer with IDD or situation.
- Questions healthcare practice when necessary for safety and quality improvement.
- Advocates for equitable healthcare consumer care.
- Informs administrators or others of the risks, benefits, and outcomes of programs and decisions that affect healthcare delivery.
- Respects the right of the healthcare consumer with IDD to self-determination and inclusion the healthcare consumer in decisions unless the healthcare consumer's incapacity to participate in a specific decision is demonstrated. Family or a legally designated guardian is included in decision-making or makes the decision as a surrogate decision-maker if legally required.
- Identifies a surrogate for healthcare decisions in lieu of a formal guardianship process, when appropriate and in accordance with local or state statutes.
- Advocates for the healthcare consumer with IDD in self-determination decisions when in conflict with the surrogate decision-maker.

- Facilitates the self-determination decisions of the healthcare consumer with IDD in all healthcare settings.
- Acts as an advocate for the healthcare consumer with IDD and family or legal guardians and initiates referral to a qualified advocate for healthcare consumers with IDD when appropriate.
- Works to prevent abuse or exploitation of the healthcare consumer with IDD and promptly responds to suspicion or evidence by reporting to appropriate authorities.
- Assists in assuring that the living arrangement for the healthcare consumer with IDD is the most appropriate and inclusive environment.
- Contributes to the educational program recommendations and advocates for inclusive environments to maximize the potential of the healthcare consumer with IDD.
- Contributes to the life plan via advocacy for the most appropriate employment situation for the healthcare consumer with IDD. The nurse assists in identifying reasonable accommodations to maximize the healthcare consumer's performance and satisfaction with chosen employment.
- Assists in the referral process for local, state, regional, and federal assistance programs.
- Supports the expression of sexuality of the healthcare consumer with IDD in a manner that is consistent with the healthcare consumer's native culture, gender preference, religious upbringing, family values, and level of maturity and provides counseling as appropriate.
- Contributes to an environment that protects the healthcare consumer with IDD from sexual exploitation at home, school, work, and community.
- Serves as an advocate to ensure that the healthcare consumer with IDD receives coordinated, continuous, and accessible health care that is provided by a professional who is competent in managing health concerns of healthcare consumers with IDD and family or legal guardians.

- Provides or arranges for effective and appropriate palliative care for healthcare consumers with IDD who undergo tests or treatments for illnesses, have chronic conditions, or are at the end of life.
- Advocates for life-sustaining treatment or refusal/withdrawal of life-sustaining treatment as the healthcare consumer with IDD and family or legal guardians decide.
- Provides support and resources for end-of-life care, grief, and bereavement when healthcare consumers with IDD experience loss.
- Participates in interprofessional teams that include family team members that address ethical risks, benefits, and outcomes.
- Advances the profession through research and scholarly inquiry, professional standards development, and influencing the generation of both nursing and health policy.
- Collaborates with other health professionals and the public to protect human rights, promote health diplomacy, and reduce health disparities for the healthcare consumer with IDD and their family or legal guardians.
- Articulates nursing values in work with professional organizations.
- Maintains the integrity of the profession.
- Integrates principles of social justice into nursing and health policy on behalf of consumers with IDD, their families, and legal guardians.

ADDITIONAL COMPETENCIES FOR THE APRN WHO SPECIALIZES IN IDD

The APRN who specializes in IDD:

- Informs the healthcare consumer with IDD and family or legal guardians of the risks, benefits, and outcomes of healthcare regimens to allow informed decision-making, including informed consent and informed refusal.

STANDARD 8. CULTURALLY CONGRUENT PRACTICE

The registered nurse who specializes in IDD practices in a manner that is congruent with cultural diversity and inclusion principles, especially as it relates to individuals with IDD.

Competencies
The IDD registered nurse:

- Demonstrates respect, equity, and empathy in actions and interactions with all healthcare consumers with IDD and families or legal guardians.
- Participates in lifelong learning to understand cultural preferences, worldview, choices, and decision-making processes of diverse consumers with IDD and their families or legal guardians.
- Creates an inventory of one's own values, beliefs, and cultural heritage.
- Applies knowledge of variations in health beliefs, practices, and communication patterns in all nurse practice activities.
- Identifies the stage of the consumer's acculturation and accompanying patterns of needs and engagement.
- Considers the effects and impact of discrimination and oppression on practice within and among vulnerable cultural groups.
- Uses skills and tools that are appropriately vetted for the culture, literacy, and language of the population with IDD and their families or legal guardians served.
- Communicates with appropriate language and behaviors, including the use of medical interpreters and translators and assistive devices in accordance with preferences of consumer with IDD and family or legal guardians.
- Identifies the cultural-specific meaning of interactions, terms, and content.
- Respects consumer with IDD decisions based on age, tradition, belief and family influence, and stage of acculturation.

- Advocates for policies that promote health and prevent harm among culturally diverse, underserved, or underrepresented consumers with IDD and their families or legal guardians.
- Promotes equal access for consumers with IDD and families or legal guardians to services, tests, interventions, health promotion programs, enrollment in research, education, and other opportunities.
- Educates nurse colleagues and other professionals about cultural similarities and differences of healthcare consumers with IDD, families or legal guardians, groups, communities, and populations.

ADDITIONAL COMPETENCIES FOR THE GRADUATE-LEVEL PREPARED REGISTERED NURSE

In addition to the competencies of the registered nurse, the graduate-level prepared registered nurse who specializes in IDD:

- Evaluates tools, instruments, and services provided to culturally diverse populations.
- Advances organizational policies, programs, services, and practices that reflect respect, equity, and values for diversity and inclusion of consumers with IDD and families or legal guardians.
- Engages consumers with IDD, families or legal guardians, key stakeholders, and others in designing and establishing internal and external cross-cultural partnerships.
- Conducts research to improve health care and healthcare outcomes for culturally diverse consumers with IDD and their families or legal guardians.
- Develops recruitment and retention strategies to achieve a multicultural workforce.

ADDITIONAL COMPETENCIES FOR THE APRN

In addition to the competencies of the registered nurse and graduate-level prepared registered nurse, the APRN who specializes in IDD:

- Promotes shared decision-making solutions in planning, prescribing, and evaluating processes when the healthcare

consumers with IDD and their families or legal guardians' cultural preferences and norms may create incompatibility with evidence-based practice.
- Leads interprofessional teams to identify the cultural and language needs of the consumer with IDD and family or legal guardians.

STANDARD 9. COMMUNICATION

The registered nurse who specializes in IDD communicates effectively in a variety of formats in all areas of practice.

Competencies
The IDD registered nurse:

- Conveys information to healthcare consumers, families or legal guardians, the interprofessional team, and others in communication formats that promote accuracy, health literacy, and in the native language of non-English speakers.
- Discloses observations or concerns related to hazards and errors in care or the practice environment to the appropriate level of professional and institutional oversight and regulation.
- Establishes communication with other providers to minimize risks associated with forthcoming and actual transfers and transition in care delivery.
- Contributes her or his own professional perspectives in discussions pertaining to the care of individuals with IDD and their families or legal guardians with the interprofessional team.
- Uses current knowledge of the adaptive and communication skills of the healthcare consumer with IDD to communicate effectively with the healthcare consumer.
- Facilitates communication between the healthcare consumer with IDD, family or legal guardians, and members of the interprofessional team, building on the adaptive and communication strengths of the healthcare consumer with IDD.

- Confers with interdisciplinary team members, including speech and language specialists and audiologists, and family team members on the need of the individual with IDD to use assistive devices and hearing aids for communication.

STANDARD 10. COLLABORATION

The registered nurse who specializes in IDD engages in shared decision-making with the healthcare consumer with IDD, family or legal guardians, and other key stakeholders in the conduct of nursing practice.

Competencies
The IDD registered nurse:

- Partners with others to effect change and produce positive, person-centered and family-centered outcomes through the sharing of IDD knowledge of the healthcare consumer with IDD, the family or legal guardians, or situation.
- Communicates with the healthcare consumer with IDD, family or legal guardians, members of the interprofessional team, healthcare providers, and community providers regarding healthcare consumer care and the nurse's role in the provision of IDD care.
- Promotes conflict management and engagement within the professional scope of practice.
- Participates in building consensus or resolving conflict in the context of patient care for individuals with IDD and their families or legal guardians.
- Applies group process and negotiation techniques with the healthcare consumer with IDD, the family or legal guardians, and colleagues.
- Adheres to standards and applicable codes of conduct that govern behavior among peers and colleagues to create a work environment that promotes cooperation, respect, and trust.
- Cooperates in creating a documented person- and family-centered plan focused on outcomes and decisions related to care

and delivery of services that indicates communication and involvement with healthcare consumers with IDD, families or legal guardians, and others.
- Engages in teamwork and team-building processes for the provision of person-centered and family-centered care for individuals with IDD and their families or legal guardians.
- Partners with other disciplines to enhance the outcomes of person-centered and family-centered care of healthcare consumers with IDD through interprofessional activities, such as education, consultation, management, technological development, continuous quality improvement, or research opportunities.
- Documents plans, communications, rationales for person-centered/family-centered plan changes, and collaborative discussions with the individual with IDD, the family or legal guardians, and interprofessional and nursing colleagues.
- Partners with the healthcare consumer with IDD and family or legal guardians or significant others to support the efforts of healthcare consumers and family or legal guardians to make appropriate decisions about utilization and allocation of resources.

ADDITIONAL COMPETENCIES FOR THE APRN WHO SPECIALIZES IN IDD

In addition to the competencies of the registered nurse, the APRN who specializes in IDD:

- Partners with other disciplines to enhance the care of healthcare consumers with IDD through interprofessional activities, such as education, consultation, management, technological development, continuous quality improvement, or research opportunities.
- Invites the contribution of the healthcare consumer with IDD, family or legal guardians, and interprofessional and nursing team members in order to achieve optimal person- and family-centered outcomes.

- Leads in establishing, improving, and sustaining collaborative interprofessional and interagency relationships to achieve safe, quality, evidence-based health care.
- Documents communications regarding the person-centered and family-centered plan of care, rationales for changes to the plan, and collaborative interprofessional and individual with IDD, family or legal guardians' discussions to improve the care of healthcare consumers with IDD.
- Partners with other interprofessional administrative team members in policymaking and in overall agency and community planning, implementation, and evaluation of services to and programs for healthcare consumers with IDD and their families or legal guardians.

STANDARD 11. LEADERSHIP

The registered nurse who specializes in IDD leads in the professional practice setting and the profession.

Competencies

The IDD registered nurse:

- Oversees the nursing care given by others while retaining accountability for the quality of person-centered and family-centered care given to the healthcare consumer with IDD and the family or legal guardian.
- Abides by the vision, the associated goals, and the person-centered plan to implement and measure progress of a healthcare consumer with IDD or progress within the context of the healthcare organization.
- Demonstrates a commitment to continuous, lifelong learning and education for self and others in IDD and related fields.
- Mentors interprofessional and nursing colleagues for the advancement of IDD interprofessional and nursing practice, the

profession, and quality health care for individuals with IDD, their families or guardians.
- Develops communication and conflict resolution skills.
- Participates in nursing and IDD professional organizations.
- Participates in efforts to influence healthcare policy involving healthcare consumers with IDD, their families or legal guardians, and the IDD and nursing profession.
- Influences institutional, professional, and public decision-making bodies to improve the professional practice environment and healthcare outcomes of healthcare consumers with IDD and their families or legal guardians.
- Provides direction to enhance the effectiveness of the interprofessional team that provides services to individuals with IDD and their families or legal guardians based upon a person-centered and family-centered framework of care that is evidence based.
- Interprets the role of IDD nursing for healthcare consumers with IDD, families or legal guardians, interprofessional colleagues, and policymakers.
- Promotes communication of information and advancement of the profession as it relates to nursing and the field of IDD through writing, publishing, and presentations for interprofessional and nursing professional or lay audiences.
- Designs innovations to effect change in IDD nursing practice and outcomes of care for individuals with IDD and their families or guardians.

ADDITIONAL COMPETENCIES FOR THE APRN WHO SPECIALIZES IN IDD
In addition to the competencies of the registered nurse, the APRN who specializes in IDD:

- Influences decision-making bodies to improve the professional practice environment and healthcare outcomes for healthcare consumers with IDD, their families or legal guardians.
- Promotes advanced practice nursing and role development by interpreting its role for healthcare consumers with IDD and

families or legal guardians, interprofessional colleagues, and policymakers.
- Models expert IDD nursing practice to interprofessional team members, healthcare consumers with IDD, and their families or legal guardians.
- Mentors interprofessional and nursing colleagues in the acquisition of IDD clinical knowledge, skills, abilities, and judgment.

STANDARD 12. EDUCATION

The registered nurse who specializes in IDD attains knowledge and competence that reflect current nursing practice and promotes futuristic thinking.

Competencies

The IDD registered nurse:

- Identifies learning needs based on nursing knowledge, the various roles the IDD nurse may assume, and the changing needs of the IDD population.
- Participates in ongoing educational activities related to appropriate knowledge bases and professional issues needed to provide comprehensive, consumer- and family-centered care to individuals with IDD across the life course and to the families or legal guardians.
- Demonstrates a commitment to lifelong learning in the field of IDD and related areas of practice (i.e., psychology, occupational therapy, nutrition) through self-reflection and inquiry to address ongoing learning needs and personal growth needs.
- Seeks experiences that reflect current practice to maintain knowledge, skills, abilities, and judgment in clinical practice or role performance in the field of IDD and related areas of practice (i.e., psychology, occupational therapy, nutrition).
- Acquires knowledge and skills appropriate to the IDD role, population, specialty, setting, or situation.

- Seeks formal and independent learning experiences to develop and maintain clinical and professional skills and knowledge in the field of IDD and related areas of practice (i.e., psychology, occupational therapy, nutrition).
- Participates in formal or informal IDD consultations to address issues in IDD nursing practice as an application of education, knowledge base, and evidence-based practice.
- Shares educational findings, experiences, and ideas with peers in the field of IDD and related areas of practice (i.e., psychology, occupational therapy, nutrition).
- Contributes to a work environment conducive to the education of interdisciplinary healthcare professionals and paraprofessionals.
- Maintains professional records that provide evidence of competence and lifelong learning in the field of IDD and related areas of practice (i.e., psychology, occupational therapy, nutrition) for licensure and certification purposes.
- Uses current healthcare research findings and other evidence related to the care of healthcare consumers with IDD to expand competencies pertaining to knowledge, skills, abilities, and judgment; to enhance role performance; and to increase knowledge of professional issues related to IDD nursing.

STANDARD 13. EVIDENCE-BASED PRACTICE AND RESEARCH

The registered nurse who specializes in IDD integrates evidence and research findings into practice.

Competencies

The IDD registered nurse:

- Utilizes current evidence-based nursing knowledge, including research findings generated in the IDD field and related fields, to guide practice.

- Incorporates evidence when initiating changes in IDD nursing practice.
- Participates, as appropriate to education level and position and IDD area of specialization, in the formulation of evidence-based practice through research and quality improvement.
- Shares personal or third-party IDD and related fields research findings with colleagues and peers.
- Participates, as appropriate to education level and position, in research, quality improvement, and scholarly activities (e.g., systematic literature reviews) to improve the health and health care of healthcare consumers with IDD and their families or legal guardians.
- Engages healthcare consumers with IDD and their families or legal guardians in research activities consistent with their informed consent, assent, and informed refusal.
- Solicits input and engagement from healthcare consumers with IDD and their families or legal guardians on the development and implementation of research activities.

ADDITIONAL COMPETENCIES FOR THE APRN WHO SPECIALIZES IN IDD
In addition to the competencies of the registered nurse, the APRN who specializes in IDD:

- Contributes to IDD nursing knowledge by conducting or synthesizing research, quality improvement, scholarly activities (e.g., systematic literature reviews), and other evidence that discovers, examines, and evaluates current practice, knowledge, theories, criteria, and creative approaches to improve healthcare outcomes of healthcare consumers with IDD and their families or legal guardians.
- Promotes a climate of research and clinical inquiry in the IDD field.
- Disseminates research findings through activities such as podium and poster presentations, publications, consultations, and journal clubs.

STANDARD 14. QUALITY OF PRACTICE

The registered nurse who specializes in IDD contributes to quality nursing practice.

Competencies

The IDD registered nurse:

- Demonstrates quality nursing care by documenting the application of the nursing process in a responsible, accountable, and ethical manner that is evidence based.
- Uses creativity and innovation to enhance comprehensive nursing care that is person and family centered of healthcare consumers with IDD and their families or legal guardians.
- Participates in quality improvement. Activities may include: examination of care practices in the hospital setting; implementation of intervention in community-based setting designed to prevent transmission of infections; and development of person-centered care programs.
- Provides leadership in the implementation of quality improvements for healthcare consumers with IDD and their families or legal guardians.
- Designs innovations to effect evidence-based change in practice and improve health and quality-of-life outcomes of healthcare consumers with IDD and their families.
- Participates in the programmatic evaluation of the practice environment and continuous quality improvement projects of nursing care provided to healthcare consumers with IDD and their families or legal guardians.
- Evaluates nursing care delegated to other professionals, direct care support professionals, unlicensed assistive personnel, or the family or legal guardians.
- Monitors health outcomes of the healthcare consumer with IDD in terms of measures of consumer satisfaction, measurable consumer outcomes, and costs.
- Identifies opportunities for the generation, dissemination, and use of research and evidence in IDD nursing.

- Participates in IDD and interprofessional organizations that strive to improve the quality of nursing and health care provided to healthcare consumers with IDD and their families or legal guardians.

Additional competencies for the APRN who specializes in IDD

In addition to the competencies of the registered nurse, the APRN who specializes in IDD nursing:

- Provides leadership in the design and implementation of continuous quality improvement projects.
- Evaluates, on a continual basis, the practice environment and quality of nursing care rendered to individuals with IDD and families or legal guardians in relation to existing evidence.
- Identifies opportunities for the generation, dissemination, and use of IDD research and evidence in professional and consumer forums.
- Obtains and maintains IDD professional certification, as needed.
- Uses the results of continuous quality improvement to initiate changes in IDD nursing practice and the healthcare delivery system for individuals with IDD and their families or legal guardians.

STANDARD 15. PROFESSIONAL PRACTICE EVALUATION

The registered nurse who specializes in IDD evaluates one's own and others' nursing practice in relation to professional practice standards and guidelines, relevant statutes, rules, and regulations.

Competencies

The IDD registered nurse:

- Engages in self-evaluation of practice on a regular basis, identifying areas of strength, as well as areas in which professional development in IDD and related fields would be beneficial.

- Obtains informal feedback regarding her or his own practice from healthcare consumers with IDD, family or legal guardians, peers, professional nursing and interprofessional colleagues, and others, including direct care support professionals.
- Participates in systematic peer review as appropriate.
- Takes action to achieve goals identified during the evaluation process.
- Provides the evidence for practice decisions and actions as part of the informal and formal evaluation processes.
- Interacts with peers and colleagues to enhance her or his own professional IDD nursing practice or role performance.
- Provides peers with formal or informal constructive feedback regarding their IDD practice or role performance.

ADDITIONAL COMPETENCIES FOR THE APRN WHO SPECIALIZES IN IDD
In addition to the competencies of the registered nurse, the APRN who specializes in IDD:

- Engages in a formal process seeking feedback regarding her or his own practice from healthcare consumers, peers, professional nursing and interprofessional colleagues, and others, including direct care support professionals.

STANDARD 16. RESOURCE UTILIZATION

The registered nurse specializing in IDD utilizes appropriate resources to plan, provide, and sustain evidence-based nursing services that are safe, effective, and fiscally responsible to healthcare consumers with IDD.

Competencies
The IDD registered nurse:

- Assesses healthcare consumer care needs and the resources available to achieve desired outcomes for individuals with IDD and their families or legal guardians.

- Identifies resource allocation for the needs of the healthcare consumer with IDD, desired outcome, complexity of the strategy to meet their comprehensive needs, and the potential for harm if needs are not addressed.
- Delegates elements of person-centered/family-centered care to appropriate healthcare workers in accordance with any applicable legal or policy parameters or principles.
- Identifies the evidence when evaluating resources for individuals with IDD and their families or legal guardians.
- Advocates for resources, including technology, that enhance IDD nursing practice.
- Modifies IDD nursing practice when necessary to promote positive interaction between healthcare consumers with IDD, their families or parents, care providers, and technology.
- Assists the healthcare consumer with IDD and family or legal guardians in identifying and securing appropriate services to address their needs across the healthcare continuum and life course.
- Assists the healthcare consumer with IDD and family or legal guardians in factoring costs, risks, and benefits in decisions about treatment and care.
- Applies innovative solutions and strategies to obtain appropriate resources for individuals with IDD and their families or legal guardians.
- Utilizes organizational resources to ensure a work environment that is conducive to completing the identified person-centered/family-centered plan and outcomes for individuals with IDD and their families or legal guardians.
- Designs evaluation methods that measure safety and effectiveness of person-centered/family-centered interventions and outcomes for individuals with IDD and their families or legal guardians.
- Promotes activities that assist healthcare professionals and health care and community-based providers and policymakers, as appropriate, in becoming informed about costs, risks, and benefits of care, or of the plan and solution.

- Addresses discriminatory healthcare practices and the impact on resource allocation, especially for the IDD population and their caregivers.

ADDITIONAL COMPETENCIES FOR THE APRN WHO SPECIALIZES IN IDD
In addition to the competencies of the registered nurse, the APRN who specializes in IDD:

- Utilizes organizational and community resources to formulate interprofessional person-centered/family-centered plans of care for individuals with IDD and their families or legal guardians.
- Formulates innovative solutions for healthcare consumer care for individuals with IDD and their families or legal guardians that utilize resources effectively and maintain quality of care.
- Designs evaluation strategies that demonstrate cost-effectiveness, cost benefit, and efficiency factors associated with IDD nursing practice.

STANDARD 17. ENVIRONMENTAL HEALTH

The registered nurse who specializes in IDD practices in an environmentally safe and healthy manner that promotes environmentally safe settings beneficial to the health and well-being of individuals with IDD.

Competencies
The IDD registered nurse:

- Attains knowledge of environmental health concepts, such as implementation of environmental health strategies.
- Promotes a practice environment that reduces environmental health risks for workers and healthcare consumers with IDD and their families or legal guardians.
- Assesses the practice environment for factors such as sound, odor, noise, and light that threaten health.

- Advocates for the safe, judicious, and appropriate use of products in health care.
- Communicates information about environmental health risks and exposure reduction strategies to healthcare consumers with IDD, families or legal guardians, colleagues, and communities.
- Utilizes scientific evidence to determine if a product or treatment is an environmental threat.
- Participates in strategies to promote healthy communities for individuals with IDD and their families or legal guardians.
- Identifies developmental and behavioral characteristics that predispose healthcare consumers with IDD to increased risk of exposure to environmental hazards and risks.
- Carefully assesses the home, school, and work environments of healthcare consumers with IDD and their families or legal guardians for potential threat of exposure to environmental hazards and risks.
- Uses knowledge of chronic health disorders and IDD to distinguish between signs and symptoms associated with disorders and disabilities and signs and symptoms associated with harmful environmental exposures.
- Develops strategies to prevent and minimize environmental health risks for healthcare consumers with IDD and their families and legal guardians.

ADDITIONAL COMPETENCIES FOR THE APRN WHO SPECIALIZES IN IDD

In addition to the competencies of the registered nurse, the APRN who specializes in IDD:

- Creates interagency and interprofessional partnerships that promote sustainable environmental health policies and conditions for individuals with IDD and their families or legal guardians.
- Analyzes the impact of social, political, and economic influences on the environment and human health risk exposures for

individuals with IDD across the life course and their families or legal guardians.
- Critically evaluates the manner in which environmental health issues related to the needs of individuals with IDD, their families or legal guardians are presented by the popular media.
- Advocates for implementation of environmental principles for IDD nursing practice.
- Supports IDD nurses in advocating for and implementing environmental principles in IDD nursing practice.

Glossary

Advanced practice registered nurses (APRNs). A nurse who completed an accredited graduate-level education program preparing her or him for the role of certified nurse practitioner, certified registered nurse anesthetist, certified nurse-midwife, or clinical nurse specialist; has passed a national certification examination that measures the APRN role and population-focused competencies; maintains continued competence as evidenced by recertification; and is licensed to practice as an APRN (adapted from APRN Joint Dialogue Group, 2008).

Advanced practice registered nurses (APRNs) specializing in IDD. An APRN with IDD specialization requires specialized knowledge and skills obtained through formal and continuing education (i.e., Leadership Education in Neurodevelopmental Disabilities, meeting presentations on IDD health issues) related to the health care and management of conditions that are general or unique to the IDD population and their families.

Assessment. A systematic, dynamic process by which the registered nurse, through interaction with the patient, family or legal guardians, groups, communities, populations, and healthcare providers, collects pertinent data, including but not limited to demographics, social determinants of health, health disparities, and physical, functional, psychosocial, emotional, cognitive, sexual, cultural, age-related, environmental, spiritual/transpersonal, and economical assessments in a systematic, ongoing process with compassion and respect for the inherent dignity, worth, and unique attributes of every person. This may involve observation, interviewing, and the use of screening and assessment tools. Diagnostic tests may be used as part of the assessment process if the nurse has specific training in that area (e.g., developmental diagnostic testing).

Assistive technology (AT). The application of scientific knowledge for practical purposes. Adaptive devices can be developed and used to assist individuals with IDD to improve and maintain the individual's level of functioning. They can be used to assist with all forms of activities such as the activities of daily living (ADL) that include bathing, dressing, grooming, and eating. Examples of ADL AT devices include wheelchairs, walkers, bath benches, grab bars, ramps, adaptive utensils, and long-handled devices for dressing or reaching. AT devices are used to support work-related activities and facilitate learning, such as the use of computers, workstation adaptations, automated page turners, and hearing aids.

Autonomy. The capacity of a nurse to determine her or his own actions through independent choice, including demonstration of competence, within the full scope of nursing practice.

Caregiver. A person who provides direct care (the provision of what is necessary for the health, welfare, maintenance, and protection of someone) for another, such as a child, dependent adult, or individual with a disability or chronic illness.

Code of ethics (nursing). A list of provisions that makes explicit the primary goals, values, and obligations of the nursing profession and expresses its values, duties, and commitments to the society of which it is a part. In the United States, nurses abide by and adhere to Code of Ethics for Nurses with Interpretive Statements (ANA, 2015b).

Collaboration. A professional healthcare partnership grounded in a reciprocal and respectful recognition and acceptance of: each partner's unique expertise, power, and sphere of influence and responsibilities; the commonality of goals; the mutual safeguarding of the legitimate interest of each party; and the advantages of such a relationship (ANA, 2015a).

Competency. An expected and measurable level of nursing performance that integrates knowledge, skills, abilities, and judgment, based on established scientific knowledge and expectations for nursing practice.

Comprehensive care. Care that integrates health (primary, secondary, and tertiary levels) and social or family or legal guardian support and service programs with educational or vocational services.

Continuity of care. An interprofessional process that includes healthcare consumers, families or legal guardians, and other stakeholders in the development of a coordinated plan of care. This process facilitates the healthcare consumer's transition between settings and healthcare providers, based on changing needs and available resources.

Coordinated care (also known as coordination of care). Care that facilitates access to needed resources and services and promotes continuity of care among multiple providers and diverse service systems. Work is done collaboratively with the healthcare consumer and family or legal guardians to achieve mutually agreed-upon goals. Timeliness, appropriateness, and completeness of care are central to this concept.

Cultural competence. Care that respects, honors, and incorporates beliefs, norms, attitudes, and life practices of healthcare consumers and their families or legal guardians congruent with their values and practices.

Cultural knowledge. The concepts and language of an ethnic or social group used to describe their health-related values, beliefs, and traditional practices, as well as the etiologies of their conditions, preferred treatments, and any contraindications for treatments or pharmacological interventions. Historical events, such as war-related migration, oppression, and structural discrimination, are also included, when relevant (ANA, 2015a).

Cultural skills. The integration of cultural knowledge and expertise into practice when assessing, communicating with, and providing care for members of a racial, ethnic, or social group (ANA, 2015a).

Delegation. The transfer of responsibility for the performance of a task from one individual to another while retaining accountability for the outcome. Example: The registered nurse, in delegating a task to unlicensed assistive personnel, transfers the responsibility for performance of the task but retains professional accountability for the overall care.

Developmentally appropriate care. Care, or the provision of what is necessary for the health, welfare, protection, and maintenance, and protection of someone, that is focused on the unique needs of healthcare consumers across the life course to promote developmental skills and independence congruent with the healthcare consumer's present functional abilities rather than chronological age.

Developmental disability (DD). Refers to an individual's lifelong mental or physical disability or combination of mental and physical disability manifested before age 22 that results in substantial limitations in three or more major life activities: (a) self-care; (b) receptive and expressive language; (c) learning; (d) mobility; (e) self-direction; (f) capacity for independent living; and (g) economic self-sufficiency. Some form of lifelong support is needed for activities of daily living and lifestyle pursuits.

Developmental screening. Generally assessing a person's global or specific domains of development (state of growth or advancement) for evidence of developmental deviation. The results of screening are not diagnostic; if the results reveal a possibility of delay, they must be repeated within a short period of time. If developmental delay is suspected after the repeated screening, the person should be referred for diagnosis and appropriate treatment and intervention.

Diagnosis. A clinical judgment about the healthcare consumer's response to actual or potential health conditions or needs. The diagnosis provides the basis for development and determination of a plan to achieve expected outcomes. Registered nurses use nursing and medical diagnoses depending upon educational and clinical preparation and legal authority.

Diagnostic overshadowing. Assigning a mental health diagnosis to a person with IDD because the person has IDD. Example: An adolescent with Down syndrome is "feeling down" after a breakup with a boyfriend. The adolescent's provider diagnoses depression without any assessment other than the history.

Early intervention. The provision of health, social, and educational services in an interprofessional setting for children from birth to three years of age who are at risk for or who have IDD.

Environment. The surrounding habitat, context, milieu, conditions, and atmosphere in which all living systems participate and interact. It includes the physical habitat as well as cultural, psychological, social, and historical influences. It includes both the external physical space as well as an individual's internal physical, mental, emotional, social, and spiritual experience (ANA, 2015a; AHNA & ANA, 2013).

Environmental health. Aspects of human health, including quality of life, that are determined by physical, chemical, biological, social, and psychological influences in the environment. It also refers to the theory and practice of assessing, correcting, controlling, and preventing those factors in the environment that can potentially adversely affect the health of present and future generations.

Evaluation. The process of determining the progress toward attainment of expected outcomes, including the effectiveness of care.

Evidence-based practice (EBP). A lifelong problem-solving approach that integrates the best evidence from well-designed research studies and evidence-based theories; clinical expertise and evidence from assessment of the health consumer's history and condition, as well as healthcare resources; and patient, family, group, community, and population preferences and values. When EBP is delivered in a context of caring, as well as an ecosystem or environment that supports it, the best clinical decisions are made to yield positive healthcare consumer outcomes (ANA, 2015a; Melnyk, Gallagher-Ford, Long, & Fineout-Overholt, 2014).

Expected outcomes. End results that are measurable, desirable, and observable, and translate into observable behaviors or relate to policies, funding, and organizations.

Family. Family of origin or significant others, such as legal guardians, if identified by the healthcare consumer.

Family-centered care. Care to healthcare consumers in need of special services (e.g., therapies, rehabilitation, adaptive equipment) that is provided within the context of the healthcare consumer's family. The strengths, individuality, and diversity of each family or legal guardian are acknowledged and valued. The cornerstone of family-centered care is a partnership between the families or legal guardians and the professionals.

Health. An experience that is often expressed in terms of wellness and illness and may occur in the presence or absence of disease or injury.

Healthcare consumer. The person, client, family, group, community, or population who is the focus of attention and to whom the registered nurse is providing services as sanctioned by the state regulatory bodies.

Healthcare providers. Individuals with special expertise who provide healthcare services or assistance to healthcare consumers with IDD. They may include nurses, physicians, psychologists, social workers, nutritionists/dietitians, and various therapists.

Health home (Medical home). Care that uses primary care providers to ensure the delivery of coordinated, comprehensive care.

Illness. The subjective experience of discomfort, disharmony, or imbalance. Not synonymous with disease.

Implementation. Activities such as teaching, monitoring, providing, counseling, delegating, and coordinating.

Inclusion. Integration of all persons, regardless of special needs and disabilities or the environment (e.g., school, community, etc.), with typical peers in the least restrictive setting. Innovative programs geared to the healthcare consumer's strengths and capabilities must be provided.

Individualized education plan (IEP). An annual educational program plan and goals that are jointly determined by the school teachers, therapists, school nurse, and parents of the school-aged child with IDD and members of their support system. The IEP includes all developmental and academic testing results, the child's health status, and the child's strengths and weaknesses, as well as transition plans. This plan may include vocational goals beginning at age 14 and is known as the individualized transition plan.

Individualized family service plan (IFSP). A program, usually developed annually and updated as needed, for the identified related group, or family, that includes goals and interventions for the entire family of a child, aged birth to three years, with or at risk for an IDD. The IFSP includes the child's strengths and weaknesses, the results of developmental testing in all areas of adaptive living, family needs, the identification of community resources, and transitional plans to the school setting. This plan is devised by the interprofessional team and the parents or legal guardians of the child with IDD and members of their support system.

Individualized plan for employment (IPE). A work or habilitation plan is completed annually for adults with IDD and includes goals and interventions as determined by the healthcare consumer, his or her family or legal guardians, and the interprofessional team at the healthcare consumer's place of employment or residence. The IPE includes all developmental, adaptive skill levels, habilitative training and skill levels, and the healthcare consumer's strengths and weaknesses, which are summarized in the plan.

Individualized transition plan (ITP). The ITP is for high school students. An ITP is an annual program developed to plan for school to post-school transition (the process of changing from one state to another), to begin when the adolescent with IDD becomes 14–16 years of age. Includes goals and interventions as determined by the healthcare consumer, his or her family or legal guardians, and the interprofessional team for the transition to adulthood. The ITP also includes the healthcare consumer's health, developmental, and adaptive skill levels, strengths and weaknesses, and goals for a successful transition into adulthood that incorporates all aspects of the healthcare consumer's life.

Information. Data that are interpreted, organized, or structured.

Intellectual and developmental disability nursing. IDD nursing focuses on protecting, promoting, and optimizing the health and functioning ability of persons with IDD; diagnosing and treating persons with IDD to maximize their quality of life and alleviate discomfort and suffering; and advocating for and with persons with IDD and their families within and across groups, communities, and society.

Intellectual disability. Refers to an individual's lifelong mental disability, manifested before age 22 that results in substantial limitations in three or more major life activities: (a) self-care; (b) receptive and expressive language; (c) learning; (d) mobility; (e) self-direction; (f) capacity for independent living; and (g) economic self-sufficiency. Some form of lifelong support is needed for activities of daily living and lifestyle pursuits.

Interprofessional. Reliant on the overlapping knowledge, skills, and abilities of each professional team member, resulting in synergistic effects by which outcomes are enhanced and become more comprehensive than a simple aggregation of the individual efforts of the team members.

Interprofessional collaboration. Integrated enactment of knowledge, skills, and values/attitudes that define working together across the professions, with other healthcare workers, and with patients, along with families and communities, as appropriate to improve health outcomes (IECEP, 2011).

Interprofessional team. A group of professionals with varied and specialized backgrounds who work with the healthcare consumer and family or legal guardians to make decisions about all aspects of the life of the healthcare consumer with IDD, including health, education, and vocational needs. This planning should be person-centered. The membership of the interprofessional team should be determined by the type of expertise needed to meet the healthcare consumer's needs.

Least restrictive environment (LRE). The environment that offers the person with IDD the least amount of restriction in carrying out activities of daily living.

Motion analysis. The analysis or examination of the elements of the process of moving. Motion analysis captures video of human motion with specialized computer software that analyzes the motion in detail. The technique gives healthcare providers a detailed picture of a person's specific movement challenges to guide proper therapy.

Musculoskeletal modeling and simulations. These computer simulations of the human body can pinpoint underlying mechanical problems in a person with a movement-related disability. This technique can help improve assistive aids or physical therapies.

Normalization. Providing a supportive environment for healthcare consumers with IDD to make decisions regarding activities of daily living and to live as close as possible to the norms and patterns in the mainstream of the society in which they reside. If this is not possible, then supporting the family or legal guardians who care for the healthcare consumer with IDD.

Nursing. The protection, promotion, and optimization of health and abilities; prevention of illness and injury; facilitation of healing; alleviation of suffering through the diagnosis and treatment of human response to health and illness; and advocacy in the care of individuals, families or legal guardians, communities, and populations.

Nursing practice. The collective professional activities of nurses, characterized by the interrelations of human responses, theory application, nursing actions, and outcomes.

Nursing process. A critical thinking model used by nurses that comprises the integration of the singular, concurrent actions of these six components: assessment, diagnosis, identification of outcomes, planning, implementation, and evaluation.

Patient. See Healthcare consumer.

Peer review. A collegial, systematic, and periodic process by which registered nurses are held accountable for practice, and that fosters the refinement of a nurse's knowledge, skills, and decision-making at all levels and in all areas of practice.

Person-centered care. Care (the provision of what is necessary for the health, welfare, maintenance, and protection of someone) that is focused on the wishes of the healthcare consumer with IDD after the healthcare consumer (and the healthcare consumer's family or legal guardians) is fully informed of the knowledge and options available regarding his or her care.

Plan. A comprehensive outline of the components that must be addressed to attain expected outcomes.

Quality. The degree to which health services for patients, families or legal guardians, groups, communities, or populations increase the likelihood of desired outcomes and are consistent with current professional knowledge.

Registered nurse. An individual registered or licensed by a state, commonwealth, territory, government, or other regulatory body to practice as a registered nurse.

Robotics. Specialized robots help regain and improve function in arms or legs after a stroke.

Scope of Nursing Practice. The description of the who, what, where, when, why, and how of nursing practice that addresses the range of nursing practice activities common to all registered nurses. When considered in conjunction with Standards of Professional Nursing Practice (2015a) and Code of Ethics for Nurses (2015b), comprehensively describes the competent level of nursing common to all registered nurses.

Standards. Authoritative statements defined and promoted by the profession by which the quality of practice, service, or education can be evaluated.

Standards of Practice. Describe a competent level of nursing care as demonstrated by the nursing process. See also Nursing process.

Standards of Professional Nursing Practice. Authoritative statements of the duties that all registered nurses, regardless of role, population, or specialty, are expected to perform competently.

Standards of Professional Performance. Describe a competent level of behavior in the professional role.

Surrogate. A consumer-designated or legally designated individual to serve on behalf of the individual as the decision-maker for health care and other lifestyle decisions (i.e., housing). Also known as a proxy.

Transcranial direct current stimulation (tDCS). In tDCS, a mild electrical current travels through the skull and stimulates the brain. This can help recover movement in patients recovering from stroke or other conditions.

Transcranial magnetic stimulation (TMS). TMS sends magnetic impulses through the skull to stimulate the brain. This system can help people who have had a stroke recover movement and brain function.

Transition. Refers to the passage from a stage of development, service system of care to another. The transition requires the individual to prepare for the change, learn new skills and knowledge needed to make the change, and adapt to the new set of circumstances.

Virtual reality. People who are recovering from injury can retrain themselves to perform motions within a virtual environment.

Wellness. Integrated, congruent functioning aimed toward reaching one's highest potential (AHNA & ANA, 2013; ANA, 2015a).

References

Acharya, K., Schindler, A., & Heller, T. (2016). Aging: Demographics, trajectories, and health system issues. In L. Rubin, J. Merrick, D. Greydanus, & D. Patel (Eds.), *Health care for people with intellectual and developmental disabilities across the lifespan* (3rd ed., pp. 1423–1432). Basel, Switzerland: Springer Publishing.

Advanced Practice Registered Nurses Joint Dialogue Group. (2008, July 7). *Consensus model for APRN regulation: Licensure, accreditation, certification & education*. Retrieved from http://www.nursingworld.org/ConsensusModelforAPRN.

Agency for Healthcare Research and Quality. (n.d.) *TeamSTEPPS: Strategies and tools to enhance performance and patient safety*. Retrieved from http://www.ahrq.gov/professionals/education/curriculum-tools/teamstepps/

Aggen, R. L., DeGennaro, M. D., Fox, L., Hahn, J. E., Logan, B.A., & VonFumetti, L. (1995). *Standards of developmental disabilities nursing practice*. Eugene, OR: Developmental Disabilities Nurses Association.

Aggen, R. L., & Moore, N. J. (1984). *Standards of nursing practice in mental retardation/developmental disabilities*. Albany, NY: New York State Office of Mental Retardation and Developmental Disabilities.

Al-Motlaq, M. A., Carter, B., Neill, S., Hallstrom, I. K., Foster, M., Coyne I, … Shields, L. (2018). Toward developing consensus on family centered care: An international descriptive study and discussion. *Journal of Child Health Care*. Retrieved from https://doi.org/10.1177/1367493518795341

American Association of Colleges of Nursing (AACN). (2019). *Fact sheet: Degree completion programs for registered nurses: RN to Master's degree and RN to baccalaureate programs*. Washington, DC: Author. Retrieved May 12, 2019, from https://www.aacnnursing.org/Portals/42/News/Factsheets/Degree-Completion-Factsheet.pdf

American Association of Colleges of Nursing (AACN). (2008). *The essentials of baccalaureate education for professional nursing practice*. Washington, DC: Author.

American Association of Colleges of Nursing (AACN). (1995). *Interdisciplinary education and practice*. Retrieved from https://www.aacnnursing.org/News-Information/Position-Statements-White-Papers/Interdisciplinary-Education-Practice

American Academy of Pediatrics. (2013). *Vaccine evidence: Examine the evidence*. Retrieved July 31, 2018, from https://www.healthychildren.org/English/safety-prevention/immunizations/Pages/Vaccine-Studies-Examine-the-Evidence.aspx

American Academy of Pediatrics (AAP), American Academy of Family Physicians (AAFP), American College of Physicians (ACP), & American Society of Internal Medicine. (2002). A consensus statement on health care transitions for young adults with special health care needs. *Pediatrics, 110,* 1304–1306.

American Association of Critical Care Nurses. (2016). *AACN standards for establishing and sustaining healthy work environments: A journey to excellence* (2nd ed.). Aliso Viejo, CA: Author.

American Association on Intellectual and Developmental Disabilities (AAIDD) Board of Directors, The Arc of the United States (Arc) Board of Directors, and Chapters of The Arc. (2018). *Self-determination.* Retrieved from https://aaidd.org/news-policy/policy/position-statements/self-determination

American Foundation for the Blind. (n.d.). *Screen readers and text-to-speech synthesizers.* Retrieved October 8, 2018, from http://www.afb.org/info/for-employers/accommodations-for-workers-with-vision-loss/screen-readers-and-text-to-speech-synthesizers/345

American Holistic Nurses Association, & American Nurses Association (ANA). (2013). *Holistic nursing: Scope & standards of practice* (2nd ed.). Silver Springs, MD: ANA.

American Nurses Association (ANA). (2019). *ANA's principles for nurse staffing* (3rd ed.). Silver Spring, MD: Author.

American Nurses Association (ANA). (2015a). *Nursing: Scope and standards of practice* (3rd ed.). Silver Spring, MD: Author.

American Nurses Association (ANA). (2015b). *Code of ethics for nurses with interpretative statements.* Silver Spring, MD: Author.

American Nurses Association (ANA). (2014a). *Addressing nurse fatigue to promote safety and health: Joint responsibilities of registered nurses and employers to reduce risks.* Retrieved from https://www.nursingworld.org/practice-policy/nursing-excellence/official-position-statements/id/addressing-nurse-fatigue-to-promote-safety-and-health/

American Nurses Association (ANA). (2014b). *Professional role competence position statement.* Retrieved December 3, 2018, from https://www.nursingworld.org/practice-policy/nursing-excellence/official-position-statements/id/professional-role-competence/

American Nurses Association (ANA). (2013a). *Public health nursing: Scope and standards of practice* (2nd ed.). Silver Springs, MD: Author.

American Nurses Association (ANA). (2013b). *Framework for measuring nurses' contributions to care coordination.* Retrieved from https://www.nursingworld.org/~4afbd6/globalassets/practiceandpolicy/health-policy/framework-for-measuring-nurses-contributions-to-care-coordination.pdf

American Nurses Association (ANA). (2013c). *Safe patient handling and mobility: Interprofessional national standards across the care continuum.* Silver Spring, MD: Author.

American Nurses Association (ANA). (2013d). *Healthy Nurse*™ Retrieved from http://www.nursingworld.org/MainMenuCategories/WorkplaceSafety/Healthy-Nurse

American Nurses Association (ANA). (2019). *ANA's principles of nurse staffing.* Silver Spring, MD: Author.

American Nurses Association (ANA). (2010a). *Nursing's social policy statement: The essence of the profession.* Silver Spring, MD: Author.

American Nurses Association (ANA). (2010b) *ANA's principles for nursing documentation: Guidance for registered nurses.* Silver Springs, MD: Author

American Nurses Association (2007). *ANA's Principles of environmental health for nursing practice with implementation strategies.* Silver Springs, MD: Author.

American Nurses Association (ANA). (2003). *Nursing's social policy statement* (2nd ed.). Silver Spring, MD: Author.

American Nurses Association (ANA). (1995). *Nursing's social policy statement.* Washington, DC: Author.

American Nurses Association (ANA). (1980). *Nursing: A social policy statement.* Kansas City, MO: Author.

American Nurses Association (ANA). (n.d.) *Healthy Nurse, Healthy Nation.* Retrieved March 27, 2019, from https://www.nursingworld.org/practice-policy/work-environment/health-safety/healthy-nurse-healthy-nation/

American Nurses Association Consensus Committee. (1994). *Standards of nursing practice for the care of children and adolescents with special health and developmental needs.* Lexington, KY: University of Kentucky, College of Nursing.

American Nurses Association Consensus Committee. (1993). *National standards of nursing practice for early intervention services.* Lexington, KY: University of Kentucky, College of Nursing.

American Psychiatric Nurses Association, International Society of Psychiatric-Mental Health Nurses, & American Nurses Association (ANA). (2014). *Psychiatric-mental health nursing: Scope and standards of practice* (2nd ed.). Silver Springs, MD: ANA.

Anderson, L., Hewitt, A., Pettingell, S., Lulinski, A., Taylor, M., & Reagan, J. (2018). *Family and Individual Needs for Disability Supports (v.2) Community Report 2017.* Minnesota: Research and Training Center on Community Living, Institute on Community Integration, University of Minnesota.

Appelgren, M., Bahsevani, C., Persson, K., & Borglin, G. (2018). Nurses' experiences of caring for patients with intellectual developmental disorders: A systematic review using a meta-ethnographic approach. *BMC Nursing,* 17(15), 1–19. Retrieved from doi.org/10.1186/s12912-018-0316-9

Auerbach, D., Staiger, D., & Buerhaus, P. (2018). Growing ranks of advanced practice clinicians — Implications for the physician workforce. *The New England Journal of Medicine, 378,* 2358–2360. Retrieved from doi.org/10.1056/NEJMp1801869

Auberry, K. (2018). Intellectual and developmental disability nursing: Current challenges in the USA. *Nursing: Research and Reviews, 8*, 23–28. Retrieved from https://doi.org/10.2147/NRR.S154511

Austin, J., Challela, M., Huber, C., Sciarillo, W., & Stade, C. (1987). *Standards for the clinical advanced practice registered nurse in developmental disabilities/handicapping conditions.* Washington, DC: American Association of University Affiliated Programs.

Barclay, A., Goulet, L. R., Holtgrewe, M. M., & Sharp, A. R. (1962). Parental evaluations of clinical services for retarded children. *American Journal on Mental Deficiency, 67*, 231–237.

Bargeron, J., Contri, D., Gibbons, L. J., Ruch-Ross, H. S., & Sanabria, K. (2015). Transition planning for youth with special health care needs (YSHCN) in Illinois schools. *Journal of School Nursing, 31*, 253–260. Retrieved from doi.org/10.1177/1059840514542130

Barnard, K. E. (1968). Teaching the retarded child is a family affair. *American Journal of Nursing, 68*, 305–311.

Barnard, K. E. (1966). Symposium on mental retardation. *Nursing Clinics of North America, 1*(4), 629–630.

Bathish, M., Wilson, C., & Potempa, K. (2018). Deliberate practice and nurse competence. *Applied Nursing Research, 40*, 106–109. Retrieved from doi.org/10.1016/j.apnr.2018.01.002. Epub 2018 Feb 3.

Bauer, L., & Bodenheimer, T. (2017). Expanded roles of registered nurses in primary care delivery of the future. *Nursing Outlook, 65*, 624–632. Retrieved from doi.org/10.1016/j.outlook.2017.03.011

Benner, P. (1984). *From novice to expert: Excellence and power in clinical nursing practice.* Menlo Park, CA: Addison-Wesley.

Betz, C. L. (2017). SPN position statement: Transition of pediatric patients into adult care. *Journal of Pediatric Nursing, 35*, 160–164. Retrieved from https://doi.org/10.1016/j.pedn.2017.05.003

Betz, C. L., Krajicek, M., & Craft-Rosenberg, M. (Eds.). (2018). *Nursing excellence in the care of children, youth and families* (2nd ed.). New York: Springer Publishing Inc.

Betz, C. L., & Nehring, W. M. (Eds.). (2010). *Nursing care for individuals with developmental disabilities: An integrated approach.* Baltimore, MD: Brookes.

Betz, C., Nehring, W. M., & Lobo, M. L. (2015). Transition needs of parents of adolescents and emerging adults with special health care needs and disabilities. *Journal of Family Nursing, 21*(3), 362–412.

Betz, C. L., & Sawin, K. J. (2018). Children and youth with disabilities and/or special health care needs and their families receive the full range of services. In C. L. Betz, M. J. Krajicek, & M. Craft-Rosenberg (Eds.), *Guidelines for nursing excellence in the care of children, youth and families* (2nd ed., pp. 249–263).

Bigby, C. & Beadle-Brown, J. (2018). Improving quality of life outcomes in supported accommodation for people with intellectual disability: What makes a difference? *Journal of Applied Research in Intellectual Disabilities, 31*, e182–e200. Retrieved from https://doi.org/10.1111/jar.12291

Blum, R.W., Garell, D., Hodgman, C. H., Jorissen, T. W., Okinow, N. A., Orr, D. P., & Slap, G. B. (1993). *Transition from child-centered to adult health-care systems for adolescents with chronic conditions.* A position paper of the Society for Adolescent Medicine. Journal of Adolescent Health, 14, 570–576.

Braddock, D. L., Hemp, R. E., Tanis, E. S., Wu, L., & Haffer, J. (2017). *State of the states in intellectual and developmental disabilities* (11th ed.). Denver, CO: Coleman Institute for Cognitive Disabilities.

Buerhaus, P. I., Skinner, H. I., Auerbach, D. I., & Staiger, D. O. (2017). Four challenges facing the nursing workforce in the United States. *Journal of Nursing Regulation, 8*, 40–46.

Butler, M, McCreedy, E., Schwer, N., Burgess, D., Call, K., Przedworski, J., … Kane, R. L. (2016). *Improving cultural competence to reduce health disparities* [Internet]. Rockville, MD: Agency for Healthcare Research and Quality (US); (Comparative Effectiveness Reviews, No. 170.) 2, Disability Populations. Retrieved from https://www.ncbi.nlm.nih.gov/books/NBK361117/

Byrne, G. (2018). Prevalence and psychological sequelae of sexual abuse among individuals with an intellectual disability: A review of the recent literature. *Journal of Intellectual Disabilities, 22*(3), 294–310.

Campinha-Bacote, J. (2011a). Coming to know cultural competence: An evolutionary process. *International Journal for Human Caring, 15*(3), 42–48.

Campinha-Bacote, J. (2011b). Delivering patient-centered care in the midst of a cultural conflict: The role of cultural competence. *The Online Journal of Issue in Nursing, 16*(2), Manuscript 5. Retrieved from https://ojin.nursingworld.org/MainMenuCategories/ANAMarketplace/ANAPeriodicals/OJIN/TableofContents/Vol-16-2011/No2-May-2011/Delivering-Patient-Centered-Care-in-the-Midst-of-a-Cultural-Conflict.html

Carling-Jenkins, R., Torr, J., Iacono, T., & Bigby, C. (2012). Experiences of supporting people with Down syndrome and Alzheimer's disease in aged care and family environments. *Journal of Intellectual & Developmental Disability, 37*(1), 54–60. Retrieved from https://doi.org/10.3109/13668250.2011.645473

Caruso, C. C., Baldwin, C. M., Berger, A., Chasens, E. R., Landis, C., Redeker, N.S., … Trinkoff, A. (2017). Position statement: Reducing fatigue associated with sleep deficiency and work hours in nurses. *Nursing Outlook, 65*, 766–768.

Center on Technology and Disability. (2018). *Assistive technology 101.* Retrieved September 28, 2018, from https://www.ctdinstitute.org/sites/default/files/file_attachments/CTD-AT101-V4.pdf

Centers for Medicare & Medicaid Services (CMS). (2014). Medicaid program; State plan home and community-based services, 5-year period for waivers, provider payment reassignment, and home and community-based setting requirements for community first choice (Section 1915(k) of the Act) and home and community-based services (HCBS) Waivers. *Federal register: The daily journal of the United States government, 79*(11): 2947–3039.

Charles, C., Gafni, A., & Whelan, T. (1997). Shared decision-making in the medical encounter: What does it mean? (or it takes at least two to tango). *Social Science & Medicine, 44*(5), 681–692. Retrieved from http://ovidsp.ovid.com/ovidweb.cgi?T=JS&PAGE=reference&D=med4&NEWS=N&AN=9032835

Chou, Y., Chiao, C., & Fu, L. (2011). Health status, social support, and quality of life among family carers of adults with profound intellectual and multiple disabilities (PIMD) in Taiwan. *Journal of Intellectual & Developmental Disability, 36*(1), 73–79. Retrieved from doi.org/10.3109/13668250.2010.529803

Christian, B. J. (2018). Translational research – the value of family-centered care for improving the quality of care for children and their families. *Journal of Pediatric Nursing, 31,* 342–345. Retrieved from doi.org/10.1016/j.pedn.2016.03.001

Cipriano, P. (2009). *Institute of Medicine 2010: A summary of the October 2009 forum on the future of nursing: Acute care.* Washington, DC: The National Academies Press. Retrieved from doi.org/10.17226/12855

Cipriano, P. F. (2014). Technology in transition. *The American Nurse, 46,* 3.

Cipriano, P. F. (2011). The future of nursing and health IT: The quality elixir. *Nursing Economics, 29*(5), 286–289, 282.

Cipriano, P. F., Bowles, K., Dailey, M., Dykes, P., Lamb, G., & Naylor, M. (2013). The importance of health information technology in care coordination and transitional care. *Nursing Outlook, 61*(6), 475–489.

Civil Rights Act, 42 USCS § 2000e (1964).

Delahunty, L. (2017). Understanding the nurse's role in identifying children with intellectual disability. *Nursing Children and Young People, 29,* 33–36. Retrieved from doi.org/10.7748/ncyp.2017.e863

Department of Defense. (2014). *Military Health System (MHS) and Defense Health Agency (DHA). TeamSTEPPS.* Retrieved from http://www.health.mil/Military-Health-Topics/Access-Cost-Quality-and-Safety/Quality-And-Safety-of-Healthcare/Patient-Safety/Patient-Safety-Products-And-Services/TeamSTEPPS

Developmental Disabilities Assistance and Bill of Rights Act Amendments of 2000, Pub. L, 106–402, 42 U.S.C. §§ 60000 et seq.

Devine, P. (1983). Mental retardation: An early subspecialty in psychiatric nursing. Journal of Psychiatric Nursing & Mental Health Services, 21, 21–30.

Dix, D. (1847). *The appeal of Dorothea Dix to Illinois General Assembly for better treatment of the insane.* Springfield, IL.

Dix, D. L. (1976). Memorial to the legislature of Massachusetts, 1843. In M. Rosen, G. R. Clark, & M. S. Kivitz (Eds.). *The history of mental retardation: Collected papers* (Vol. 1, pp. 1–30). Baltimore, MD: University Park Press.

Figueiredo-Ferraz, H., Grau-Alberola, E., Gil-Monte, P. R, & García-Juesas, J. A. (2012). Burnout and job satisfaction among nursing professionals, *Psicothema*, 24, 271–276.

Ford, K., Dickinson, A., Water, T., Campbell, S., Bray, L., & Carter, B. (2018). Child-centered care: Challenging assumptions and repositioning children and young people. *Journal of Pediatric Nursing, 43*, e39–e43. Retrieved from https://doi.org/10.1016/j.pedn.2018.08.012

Frey, R., Igielnik, R., & Patten, E. (2018*). How Millennials today compare with their grandparents 50 years ago. Fact tank, news in the numbers.* Pew Research Center. Retrieved December 17, 2018, from http://www.pewresearch.org/fact-tank/2018/03/16/how-millennials-compare-with-their-grandparents/

Fry, R. (2018). *Millennials projected to overtake Baby Boomers as America's largest generation. Fact tank, news in the numbers,* Pew Research Center. Retrieved December 17, 2018, from http://www.pewresearch.org/fact-tank/2018/03/01/millennials-overtake-baby-boomers/

Hahn, J. E. (2003). Addressing the need for education: Curriculum development for nurses about intellectual and developmental disabilities. *The Nursing Clinics of North America, 38,* 185–204.

Haynes, U. (1974). *Overview of the National Collaborative Infant Project.* Washington, DC: United Cerebral Palsy Association.

Haynes, U. (1968). *Guidelines for nursing standards in residential centers for the mentally retarded.* Washington, DC: United Cerebral Palsy Association.

Hewitt, A., Lightfoot, E., Bogenschutz, M., McCormick, K., Sedlezky, L. & Doljanac, R. (2010). Parental caregivers' desires for lifetime assistance planning for future supports for their children with intellectual and developmental disabilities. *Journal of Family Social Work, 13*(5), 420–434. Retrieved from doi.org/10.1080/10522158.2010.514678

Huston, C. (2013). The impact of emerging technology on nursing care: Warp speed ahead. *Online Journal of Issues in Nursing*, 18(2). Manuscript 1. Retrieved from http://www.nursingworld.org/MainMenuCategories/ANAMarketplace/ANAPeriodicals/OJIN/TableofContents/Vol-18-2013/No2-May-2013/Impact-of-Emerging-Technology.html

Individuals with Disabilities Education Improvement Act of 2004, PL 108=446. 20 U.S.C. §§ 1400 et seq.

Individuals with Disabilities Education Act of 1990, PL 101–476, 20 U.S.C. §§ 140 et seq.

Igoe, J. B., Green, P., Heim, H., Licata, M., MacDonough, G. P., & McHugh, B. A. (1980*). School nurses working with handicapped children.* Kansas City, MO: American Nurses Association.

Institute of Medicine (IOM). (2011). *The Future of nursing: Leading change, advancing health.* Washington, DC: The National Academies Press.

Institute of Medicine (IOM). (2003). *Health professions education: A bridge to quality.* Washington, DC: National Academies Press.

Institute of Medicine (IOM). (2001). *Crossing the quality chasm: A new health system for the 21st century*. Washington, DC: National Academies Press.

International Society of Nurses in Genetics, Inc. (ISONG), & American Nurses Association (ANA). (2016). *Genetics/genomics nursing: Scope and standards of practice* (2nd ed.). Silver Springs, MD: ANA.

International Society of Nurses in Genetics, Inc. (ISONG), & American Nurses Association (ANA). (2006). *Genetics-genomics nursing: Scope and standards of practice*. Silver Spring, MD: ANA.

International Society of Nurses in Genetics, Inc. (ISONG), & American Nurses Association (ANA). (1998). *Statement on the scope and standards of genetics clinical nursing practice*. Washington, DC: American Nurses Publishing.

Interprofessional Education Collaborative Expert Panel. (2011). *Core competencies for interprofessional collaborative practice: Report of an expert panel*. Washington, DC: Interprofessional Education Collaborative.

Janicki, M. P., Dalton, A. J., Henderson, C. M., & Davidson, P. W. (1999). Mortality and morbidity among older adults with intellectual disability: Health services considerations. *Disability Rehabilitation, 21*, 284–294.

Jaques, H., Lewis, P., O'Reilly, K., Wiese, M., & Wilson, N. J. (2018). Understanding the contemporary role of the intellectual disability nurse: A review of the literature. *Journal of Clinical Nursing, 27*, 3858–3871.

Jiang, J. (2018). *Millennials stand out for their technology use, but older generations also embrace digital life*, Pew Research Center. Retrieved May 12, 2019, from https://www.pewresearch.org/fact-tank/2019/09/09/us-generations-technology-use/

Kane, R. L., Shamilyan, T., Mueller, C., Duvall, S., & Wilt, T. J. (2007). Nurse staffing and quality of patient care. In *Agency for healthcare research and quality* (Publication No. 07-E005). Rockville, MD: Agency for Healthcare Research and Quality.

Kirch, D. G., & Petelle, K. (2017). Addressing the physician shortage: The peril of ignoring demography. *Journal of the American Medical Association, 317*(19):1947–1948. Retrieved from doi.org/10.1001/jama.2017.2714

Kleier, J. (2016). Adult patients with developmental disorders: Are you prepared? *Urologic Nursing; 36* (4), 161–162. Retrieved from doi.org/10.7257/1053-816X.2016.36.4.161

Krishna, A. (2018). Poison or prevention? Understanding the linkages between vaccine-negative individuals' knowledge deficiency, motivations, and active communication behaviors. *Health Communication, 33*, 1088–1096. Retrieved from doi.org/10.1080/10410236.2017.1331307

Kronk, R., Colbert, A., Smeltzer, S., & Blunt, E. (2020). Development of prelicensure nursing competencies in caring for people with disabilities through Delphi methodology. *Nurse Educator, 45*(3), E21–E25. https://doi.org/10.1097/nne.0000000000000712

Larson, S. A., Eschenbacher, H. J., Anderson, L. L., Taylor, B., Pettingell, S., Hewitt, A., … Bourne, M.L. (2017). *In-home and residential long-term supports and services for persons with intellectual or developmental disabilities: Status and trends through*

2015. Minneapolis: University of Minnesota, Research and Training Center on Community Living, Institute on Community Integration.

Lechtenberger, D. (2010). Education for All Handicapped Children Act of 1975. In C. S. Clauss-Ehlers (Ed.), *Encyclopedia of cross-cultural school psychology*. Boston, MA: Springer.

Leininger, M. M. (1988). Leininger's theory of nursing: Cultural care diversity and universality. *Nursing Science Quarterly, 1*(4), 152–160.

Leininger, M. M., & McFarland, M. R. (2002). Transcultural nursing: Concepts, theories, research and practice. McGraw-Hill Education.

Lulinski, A., Jorwic, N. T., Tanis, E. S., & Braddock, D. (2018). Rebalancing of long-term supports and services for individuals with intellectual and developmental disabilities in the United States. The State of the States in intellectual and developmental disabilities. *Data Brief, (2)*. Retrieved March 29, 2019, from https://www.colemaninstitute.org/wp-content/uploads/2018/04/SOS-Brief-2018_2_Rebalancing.pdf

Mahan, J. D., Betz, C. L., Okumura, M. J., & Ferris, M. E. (2017). Self-management and transition to adult health care in adolescents and young adults: A team process. *Pediatrics in Review, 38*(7), 305–319.

McFarland, M. R., & Wehbe-Alamah, H. B. (2015). The theory of culture care diversity and universality. In M. R. McFarland & H. B. Wehbe-Alamah (Eds.), *Leininger's culture care diversity and universality: A worldwide nursing theory* (3rd ed., p. 25). Burlington, MA: Jones and Bartlett Learning.

McNelly, P. C. (1966, December 2–6). *Operation six-pack [paper]*. Academy for Cerebral Palsy Meeting, New Orleans, LA.

Melnyk, B. M., Gallagher-Ford, L., Long, L. E., & Fineout-Overholt, E. (2014). The establishment of evidence-based practice competencies for practicing registered nurses and advanced practice nurses in real-world clinical settings: Proficiencies to improve healthcare quality, reliability, patient outcomes, and costs. *Worldviews on Evidence-Based Nursing, 11*(1), 5-15. https://doi.org/10.1111/wvn.12021

Miller, J. A. (1979). *A history of nursing at Central Wisconsin Center for the developmentally disabled*. Unpublished manuscript. Chicago, IL: University of Illinois.

Moulton, B., & King, J. S. (2010). Aligning ethics with medical decision-making: The quest for informed patient choice. *Journal of Law and Medical Ethics, 38*, 85–97. Retrieved from doi.org/10.1111/j.1748-720X.2010.00469.x

National Association of Pediatric Nurse Practitioners (NAPNAP). (2020). NAPNAP position statement on supporting the transition from pediatric to adult focused health care. *Journal of Pediatric Health Care, 34*, 390–394. Retrieved from https://doi.org/10.1016/j.pedhc.2020.03.006

National Association of School Nurses (NASN). (2019a). *Transition planning for students with healthcare needs (Position Statement)*. [Internet]. Silver Spring, MD: Author. Retrieved August 13, 2020, from https://www.nasn.org/nasn/advocacy/professional-practice-documents/position-statements/ps-transition

National Association of School Nurses (NASN). (2019b). *Special needs school nurses.* Retrieved May 29, 2019, from https://www.nasn.org/nasn/membership/current-members/sigs/membership-get-connected-snsn

National Association of School Nurses (NASN). (2018). *The role of the 21st century school nurse (Position Statement).* Silver Spring, MD: Author.

National Association of School Nurses (NASN). (2017a). *Students with chronic health conditions: The role of the school nurse (Position Statement).* Silver Spring, MD: Author.

National Association of School Nurses (NASN). (2017b) *About NASN.* Retrieved August 4, 2020, from https://www.nasn.org/nasn/about-nasn/about

National Association of School Nurses (NASN). (2014). *Transition planning for students with chronic health conditions (Position Statement).* Silver Spring, MD: Author.

National Association of School Nurses (NASN), & American Nurses Association (ANA). (2017). *School nursing: Scope and standards of practice* (3rd ed.). Silver Springs, MD: ANA. Retrieved from https://www.nasn.org/nasn/nasn-resources/professional-topics/scope-standards

National Council of State Boards of Nursing (NCSBN). (2018*). Progress and Precision: The NCSBN 2018 Environmental Scan, Journal of Nursing Regulation, 8*(4), S3–S6. Retrieved from doi.org/10.1016/S2155-8256(18)30014-0

National Council of State Boards of Nursing (NCSBN). (2005). *Meeting the ongoing challenge of continued competence.* Chicago, IL: Author. Retrieved from ncsbn.org

Needleman, J. (2015). Nurse staffing: The knowns and unknowns. *Nursing Economics, 33*(1), 5–7.

Nehring, W. M. (2010). Historical perspective and emerging trends. In C. L. Betz & W. M. Nehring (Eds*.), Nursing care for individuals with intellectual and developmental disabilities: An integrated approach* (pp. 1–17). Baltimore: Brookes Publishing.

Nehring, W. M. (Ed.). (2005). *Core curriculum for specializing in intellectual and developmental disability: A resource for nurses and other health care professionals.* Boston, MA: Jones and Bartlett.

Nehring, W. M. (1999). *A history of nursing in the field of mental retardation and developmental disabilities.* Washington, DC: American Association on Mental Retardation.

Nehring, W. M., & Lindsey, B. (2016). History of health care for people with intellectual and developmental disability. In I. L. Rubin, J. Merrick, D. E. Greydanus, & D. R. Patel (Eds.), *Health care for people with intellectual and developmental disabilities across the lifespan. Part 1* (pp. 33–46). Switzerland: Springer International Publishing.

Nickel, W. K., Weinberger, S. E., Guze, P. A., & Patient Partnership in Healthcare Committee of the American College of Physicians. (2018). Principles for patient and family partnership in care: An American College of Physicians position paper. *Annals of Internal Medicine, 169,* 796–799.

Nightingale, F. (1859). *Notes on nursing: What it is and what it is not.* London: John W. Parker and Son.

Nursing Division of the American Association on Mental Retardation & American Nurses Association. (1998). *Statement on the scope and standards for the nurse who specializes in developmental disabilities and/or mental retardation.* Washington, DC: American Nurses Publishing.

Office of Disease Prevention and Health Promotion, Office of the Assistant Secretary for Health, Office of the Secretary, & U.S. Department of Health and Human Services. (2020). Healthy People 2030: Building a healthier future for all. Retrieved August 18, 2020, from https://health.gov/healthypeople

O'Reilly, K., Lewis, P., Wiese, M., Goddard, L., Trip, H., Conder, J., ... Wilson, N. J. (2018). An exploration of the practice, policy and legislative issues of the specialist area of nursing people with intellectual disability: A scoping review. *Nursing Inquiry, 25*(4), e12258. Retrieved from https://doi.org/10.1111/nin.12258

Patja, K., Iivanainen, M., Vesala, H., Oksanen, H., & Ruoppila, I. (2000). Life expectancy of people with intellectual disability: A 35-year follow-up study. *Journal of Intellectual Disability Research, 44*(5), 591–599. Retrieved from https://doi.org/10.1046/j.1365-2788.2000.00280.x

Prouty, R. W., Alba, K., & Lakin, C. K. (2008). *Residential services for persons with developmental disabilities: Status and trends through 2007,* Research and Training Center on Community Living. Minneapolis, MN: University of Minnesota.

Quinn, B. L., & Smolinski, M. (2017). Improving school nurse pain assessment practices for students with intellectual disability. *Journal of School Nursing, 34,* 480–488. Retrieved from https://doi.org/10.1177/1059840517722591

Rehabilitation Act of 1973, PL. 93–112, 29 U.S.C. §§701, et seq.

Reiss, S., Levitan, G.W., & Szyszko, J. (1982). Emotional disturbance and mental retardation: Diagnostic overshadowing. *American Journal of Mental Deficiency, 86,* 567–574.

Robert Wood Johnson Foundation (2013*). The case for academic progression. Charting Nursing's Future.* Retrieved December 3, 2018, from https://www.rwjf.org/content/dam/farm/reports/issue_briefs/2013/rwjf407597

Rosen, D. S. (2003). Transition to adult health care for adolescents and young adults with chronic conditions. *Journal of Adolescent Health, 33,* 309–311.

Roth, S. P., & Morse, J. S. (Eds.). (1994*). A life-span approach to nursing care for individuals with developmental disabilities.* Baltimore, MD: Paul H. Brookes.

Singer, B. (2013). Perceptions of school nurses in the care of students with disabilities. *Journal of School Nursing, 29,* 329–36. Retrieved from https://doi.org/10.1177/1059840512462402

Smith, S. (2012). Nurse competence: A concept analysis. *International Journal of Nursing Knowledge, 23,* 172–182. Retrieved from https://doi.org/10.1111/j.2047-3095.2012.01225.x

Society of Pediatric Nurses (SPN), National Association of Pediatric Nurse Practitioners (NAPNAP), & American Nurses Association (ANA). (2015). *Pediatric nursing: Scope and standards of practice* (2nd ed.). Silver Springs, MD: ANA.

Stephens, T. M. & Gunther, M. E. (2016). Twitter, millennials, and nursing education research. *Nursing Education Perspectives, 37*(1), 23–27.

Sumner, G., & Spietz, A. (1994). *NCAST caregiver/parent-child interaction teaching manual.* Seattle, WA: NCAST Publications, University of Washington, School of Nursing.

Talente, G., & LeComte, J. (2013). SGIM announces the formation of the adults with complex conditions originating in childhood task force. *SGIM Forum, 36*(11), 1, 12.

The Joint Commission. (2012). *Hot topics in health care: Transitions of care: The need for a more effective approach to continuing patient care.* Oakbrook Terrace, IL: Author. Retrieved from http://www.jointcommission.org/assets/1/18/Hot_Topics_Transitions_of_Care.pdf

Thompson, R., & O'Quinn, A. (1979). *Developmental disabilities: Etiologies, manifestations, diagnoses and treatments.* New York: Oxford University Press.

Towle, A., Godolphin, W., Grams, G., & Lamarre, A. (2006). Putting informed and shared decision making into practice. *Health Expectations, 9,* 321–332.

Trip, H., Whitehead, L., Crowe, M., Mirfin-Veitch, B., & Daffue, C. (2019). Aging with intellectual disabilities in families: Navigating ever-changing seas—a theoretical model. *Qualitative health research, 29*(11), 1595–1610. https://doi.org/10.1177/1049732319845344

Trollor, J. N., Eagleson, C., Turner, B., Salomon, C., Cashin, A., Iacono, T., … Lennox, N. (2018). Intellectual disability content within pre-registration nursing curriculum: How is it taught? *Nurse Education Today, 69,* 48–52. Retrieved from doi.org/10.1016/j.nedt.2018.07.002

U.S. Census Bureau. (2017). *Population projections: 2017.* Retrieved December 17, 2018, from https://www.census.gov/programs-surveys/popproj/data/datasets.html

U.S. Department of Health and Human Services, National Institutes of Health, & Eunice Kennedy Shriver National Institute of Child Health and Human Development. (2018a). *What are some types of assistive devices and how are they used?* Retrieved May 29, 2019, from https://www.nichd.nih.gov/health/topics/rehabtech/conditioninfo/device

U.S. Department of Health and Human Services, National Institutes of Health, & Eunice Kennedy Shriver National Institute of Child Health and Human Development. (2018b). *What are some types of rehabilitative technologies?* Retrieved May 29, 2019, from https://www.nichd.nih.gov/health/topics/rehabtech/conditioninfo/use

U.S. Department of Labor, & Bureau of Labor Statistics, (2018). *Occupational employment and wages, May 2018, 29–1141 Registered Nurses.* Retrieved May 12, 2019, from https://www.bls.gov/oes/current/oes291141.htm#ind

U.S. Department of Labor, & Bureau of Labor Statistics, (2016). *Occupational outlook handbook, nurse anesthetists, nurse midwives, and nurse practitioners.* Retrieved December 3, 2018, from https://www.bls.gov/ooh/healthcare/nurse-anesthetists-nurse-midwives-and-nurse-practitioners.htm

U.S. Department of Labor, & Occupational Safety and Health Administration (OSHA). (2015). *Guidelines for preventing workplace violence for healthcare and social service workers* (No. 3148-04R). Washington, DC: DOL, OSHA. Retrieved March 27, 2019, from https://www.osha.gov/Publications/osha3148.pdf

U.S. Public Health Service. (2002). *Closing the gap: A national blueprint for improving the health of individuals with mental retardation* [Report of the Surgeon General's Conference on Health Disparities and Mental Retardation]. Washington, DC: Author.

Vanderbilt Kennedy Center for Excellence in Developmental Disabilities. (2018). *Informed consent in adults with intellectual or developmental disabilities*. Retrieved from http://iddtoolkit.vkcsites.org/general-issues/informed-consent/

Watson, J. (2012). *Human caring science: A theory of nursing* (2nd ed.). Sudbury, MA: Jones and Bartlett Learning.

Watson, J. (2008). *The philosophy and science of caring*. Boulder, CO: University Press of Colorado.

Watson, J. (1999). *Postmodern nursing and beyond*. Edinburgh, UK: Churchill Livingstone.

Wherry, J.S. (2004, September/October). The Influence of home on school success. *Principal*, 6. Retrieved from https://www.naesp.org/sites/default/files/resources/2/Principal/2004/S-Op6.pdf

White, P. H., Cooley, W. C.; Transitions Clinical Report Authoring Group, American Academy of Pediatrics, American Academy of Family Physicians, & American College of Physicians. (2018). Supporting the health care transition from adolescence to adulthood in the medical home. *Pediatrics, 142*(5), e20182587.

Xue, Y., Kannan, V., Greener, E., Smith, J., Brasch, J., Brent. A.J., & Spetz, J. (2018). Full scope-of-practice regulation is associated with higher supply of nurse practitioners in rural and primary care health professional shortage counties. *Journal of Nursing Regulation, 8*, 5–13. Retrieved from https://doi.org/10.1016/S2155-8256(17)30176-X

Ying, X., Kannan, V., Greener, E., Smith, J.A., Brasch, J., Johnson, B.A., & Spetz, J. (2018). Full scope-of-practice regulation is associated with higher supply of nurse practitioners in rural and primary care health professional shortage counties. *Journal of Nursing Regulation, 8*, 5–13. Retrieved from https://doi.org/10.1016/S2155-8256(17)30176-X

Index

A

AACN (American Association of Critical Care Nurses) 38–39
AADMD (American Academy of Developmental Medicine and Dentistry) 3
AAFP (American Academy of Family Physicians) 7
AAIDD. *See* American Association on Intellectual and Developmental Disabilities (AAIDD)
AAP (American Academy of Pediatrics) 7
abuse 90
academic consultation positions 52
access to health services 60
accountability 46–47
acculturation 92
ACP (American College of Physicians) 7
activities of daily living (ADL) 21, 85
ADA (Americans with Disabilities Act) 13, 49
ADL (activities of daily living) 21, 85
administrative positions 52
adults with IDD 25, 58, 68–69. *See also* intellectual and developmental disability (IDD)
    services for 69
    shift to adulthood 58
advanced practice registered nurses (APRNs) 7. *See also* APRNs who specialize in IDD
    advanced degrees 52–53
    special interest groups for IDD 59
advocacy 12–13, 30–31, 46, 49, 58, 90
aggregate-level data 75
aging population 60, 68
American Academy for Cerebral Palsy and Developmental Medicine 50
American Academy of Developmental Medicine and Dentistry (AADMD) 3
American Academy of Family Physicians (AAFP) 7
American Academy of Pediatrics (AAP) 7
American Association of Critical Care Nurses (AACN) 38–39
American Association on Intellectual and Developmental Disabilities (AAIDD) 3, 49, 50
American College of Physicians (ACP) 7
American Nurses Association (ANA)
    about the ix–x
        Committee on Nursing Practice Standards ix
        healthy work environments 37
        staff ix
American Society of Internal Medicine 7
Americans with Disabilities Act (ADA) 13, 49
ANA Scope and Standards of Practice 31
ANA's Principles of Nurse Staffing 36
APC (Advanced Practice Clinician) Section of the Society for Developmental and Behavioral Pediatrics (SDBP) 59
APRNs (advanced practice registered nurses) 7, 52–53, 59
APRNs who specialize in IDD
    assessment 74

APRNs who specialize in IDD (*cont.*)
    collaboration 96–97
    coordination of care 84
    culturally congruent practice 93–94
    diagnosis 75–76
    environmental health 107–108
    ethics 91
    evaluation 87
    evidence-based practice and research 101
    health teaching and health promotion 86
    implementation 82–83
    leadership 98–99
    outcomes identification 77
    planning 79–80
    professional practice evaluation 104
    quality of practice 103
    resource utilization 106
art of IDD nursing
    care and caring 19–21
    cultural components of care 21
assessment 8, 72–74
assistive technology (AT) 20, 63–64

B

baby boomer generation
    health and chronic illness 66–69
    nurses and experience 61
Barclay, A. 27
Barnard, Kathryn 27
Benner, P. 54
Betz, Cecily 27, 28
Braille 32
bullying 21

C

California's Lanterman Developmental Disabilities Services Act (1969) 49
care. *See also* coordination of care; *See also* self-care
    consultants 3, 100
    continuity of 80, 84
    culture and 21
    end-of-life 45, 91
    healthy nurses and 37
    in IDD nursing practice 19
    lifetime 57
    palliative 45, 91
    person-centered 76, 81
care process interventions 77
CART (Computer-Assisted Real Time text) 32
certification 56, 103
Children's Bureau 23
chronic health conditions 66, 107
Closing the Gap: A National Blueprint for Improving the Health of Persons with Mental Retardation 1
CME (continuing AT/RT classes) 65
Code of Ethics for Nurses with Interpretive Statements xi, 17, 29, 43–50, 48, 53, 88
collaboration 10, 28, 39–40, 95–97
communication 10, 18, 81, 97
    interprofessional 40, 84, 95
    primary care providers toolkit 32
    standards 94–95
community-based systems 69
comorbidities 18
competence 53–55
    definition of 53–54
    developmental model 54
    evaluating 55–56
competencies 11, 71
    assessment 72–74
    collaboration 95–97
    communication 94–95
    coordination of care 83–84
    culturally congruent practice 92–94
    diagnosis 74–76
    education 99–100
    environmental health 106–108
    ethics 88–91
    evaluation 86–87
    evidence-based practice and research 100–101
    health teaching and health promotion 85–86

implementation 80–83
leadership 97–99
outcomes identification 76–77
planning 77–80
professional practice evaluation 103–104
quality of practice 102–103
resource utilization 104–106
comprehensive evaluation system 34
Computer-Assisted Real Time text (CART) 32
conference workshops for IDD nurses 59
confidentiality 46, 48, 88
conflict management 95
consumer alliance and advocacy groups 85
consumer satisfaction 102
continuing AT/RT classes (CME) 65
continuing education 56, 62. *See also* education
continuity of care 80, 84
continuum of care, illness–health 2
coordination of care 9, 76, 83–84
cost and economic implications 77, 78, 106
critical thinking skills 54
cultural diversity 57
culturally congruent practice 10, 21, 76, 92–94
culture of safety 32
cyberbullying 21

D

data
  collection 72
  ongoing assessment 87
  synthesizing 73, 86
DBMH (NAPNAP SIG Developmental, Behavioral, and Mental Health) 59
DD. *See* developmental disability (DD)
DDNA. *See* Developmental Disabilities Nurses Association (DDNA)
decision-making 67–69. *See also* informed shared decision-making (ISDM); *See also* surrogate for healthcare decisions
deinstitutionalization 29, 60
delegation 81, 105
dementia 58
Developmental Disabilities Assistance and Bill of Rights Act of 2000 2, 4
Developmental Disabilities Nurses Association (DDNA) 3, 49, 50, 56
developmental disability (DD) 2. *See also* intellectual and developmental disability (IDD)
  definition of 4
  infants and young children 4
Developmentally Disabled Assistance and Bill of Rights Act 24
developmental needs 85
development, personal and professional 47, 62
diagnosis 8, 74–76, 87
diagnostic overshadowing 6
diagnostic tests 72, 74
differential diagnosis 75
digital natives 65
dignity of risk 45
discrimination 13, 92, 106
diversity, cultural 57, 92
Dix, Dorothea 26
Doctor of Nursing Practice (DNP) degree 51
Doctor of Philosophy (PhD) degree 51
documentation 79, 81, 87, 102
durable medical equipment 64

E

education 99–100. *See also* lifelong learning
  children with IDD 24
  continuing 56, 62
  graduate level 51–52
  health 85–86
  healthy nurse 37
  nursing 10, 51–53, 61–62
  safe patient handling 33
  technology 64–65
end-of-life care 45, 91

Enhanced Nursing Licensure Compact (eNLC) 53
environmental health 10, 106–108
environmental modifications 64
ergonomic design 33
ethics 9, 88–91
    code of 44
    interprofessional teams and 39
evaluation 9, 86–87
    of competence 55–56
    of patient outcomes 29
    of safe patient handling 34
Every Student Succeeds Act 49
evidence-based practice and research 10, 28–29, 100–101
    assessment 73
    competencies 55
    implementation 82
    planning 78
exploitation 90

F

faculty positions 52
family
    dynamics 73
    informed shared decision-making and 67–68, 96
    parents of adult children with IDD 67
    plan of care and 2, 77–79, 95
    self-determination and 19, 89
Family-Centered Care (FCC) 67
fatigue 34–35
FCC. *See* Family-Centered Care (FCC)
feedback, formal and informal 104

G

generational changes 65
generation shift 61
gene therapy 20–21
genetic and genomic health care 20–21, 58
Genetics-Genomics Nursing: Scope and Standards of Practice xii
graduate level nursing education 51–52
graduate-level prepared registered nurse who specializes in IDD
    assessment 74
    coordination of care 84
    culturally congruent practice 93
    diagnosis 75
    evaluation 87
    health teaching and health promotion 86
    implementation 81–82
    outcomes identification 77
    planning 79
The Guidelines for Nursing Standards in Residential Centers for the Mentally Retarded 24

H

Haynes, Una H. 27
healthcare
    delivery system reform 60
    financing 61
    shortage of workers 52
healthcare information technology (HIT) 63
Health Care Quality and Outcomes Guidelines for Nursing of Children, Adolescents, and Families 55
health diplomacy 91
health disparities 91
health information resources 86
health policy 61, 98
health professional shortages 52–53, 58
health services, access to 60–61
health teaching and health promotion 9, 85–86
healthy lifestyles 85
Healthy Nurse 37–38
Healthy Nurse, Healthy Nation Initiative, Code of Ethics for Nurses with Interpretive Statements 48
Healthy People 2030: People with Disabilities 41, 72
HIT (healthcare information technology) 63
human element in practice 63
human rights 91

I

IDD. *See* intellectual and developmental disability (IDD)
IDD nursing. *See* intellectual and developmental disability (IDD) nursing
IDEIA (Individuals with Disabilities Education Improvement Act) 13–14
ID (intellectual disability) 2
IECEP (Interprofessional Education Collaborative Expert Panel) 39–40
IEP (Individual Education Plans) 14, 57
IEP (Individualized Educational Program) 7
IFSP. *See* Individualized Family Service Plan (IFSP)
illness–health continuum of care 2
implementation 9, 80–83
incivility 35–36, 48
inclusion 92
Individual Education Plans (IEP) 14, 57
Individualized Educational Program (IEP) 7
Individualized Family Service Plan (IFSP) 7
Individuals with Disabilities Education Improvement Act (IDEIA) 13–14
Individual Transition Plans (ITP) 14, 57
information technology (IT) 58
informed shared decision-making (ISDM) 67–68, 76, 83
institutionalization 22–23, 29
Intellectual and Developmental Disabilities Nursing: Scope and Standards of Practice xi, 69–70
    about ix
    audience xiii
intellectual and developmental disability (IDD) 1. *See also* adults with IDD; *See also* intellectual and developmental disability (IDD) nursing
    biopsychosocial issues 2–3
    terminology, offensive 22, 24
intellectual and developmental disability (IDD) nursing
    advancement of 48–49
    art of 18–21
    competence 53–55
    definition of 2–5, 11–14
    development and function of standards 8–11
    high-performing interprofessional teams 39–40
    history of 1, 22–26
    personal and prefessional development 47
    professional trends and issues 57–70
    science of 22–29
    scope of practice 3–5, 69–70
    specialty practice 5–7
    statistical snapshot 50–51
intellectual disability (ID) 2. *See also* intellectual and developmental disability (IDD)
intergenerational differences 67
International Association for the Scientific Study of Intellectual Disability 50
internships in nursing 56
interprofessional collaboration 28, 39 40, 43, 80, 96–97, 98
interprofessional education 62
Interprofessional Education Collaborative Expert Panel (IECEP) 39–40
interprofessional providers 12
ISDM. *See* informed shared decision-making (ISDM)
IT (information technology) 58
ITP (Individual Transition Plans) 14, 57

J

journal clubs 101

K

Kennedy, John F. 14, 22
knowledge
    science of IDD nursing 22–26
    synthesizing 73, 86

L

language, native 94
leadership 10, 69, 82, 97–99
leadership education in neurodevelopmental and related disabilities (LEND) 51
least restrictive environment (LRE) 46, 49, 78. *See also* living conditions
legislation, federal and state 13–15, 48–49
LEND (Leadership Education in Neurodevelopmental and Related Disabilities) 51
licensed practical nurse (LPN) 53
licensed vocational nurse (LVN) 53
licensure and education 51–53
    competency 55–56, 100
    educational options 51
life expectancy 66
lifelong learning 54, 92, 99. *See also* education
Life-Span Approach to Nursing Care for Individuals with Developmental Disabilities 25
lifetime assistance model 67
lifetime care 57
literature reviews 101
living conditions 46. *See also* least restrictive environment (LRE)
LPN (licensed practical nurse) 53
LRE. *See* least restrictive environment (LRE)
LVN (licensed vocational nurse) 53

M

Maternal and Child Health Bureau 51
McNelly, Pat 27
medical equipment, durable 64
mental retardation. *See* intellectual and developmental disability (IDD)
mentors 97, 99
millennial generation
    nurses 61
    redefining health and well-being 65–66
Miller, J. A. 27
Mimosa Project 27

N

NAPNAP SIG Developmental, Behavioral, and Mental Health (DBMH) 59
National Association of School Nurses (NASN) 6
    NASN Special Needs School Nurses Special Interest Group 50–51
    position statements 28
negotiation 95
Nehring, W. M. 28
Nixon, Richard 24
nurse internships 56
Nurse's Role in Providing Ethically and Developmentally Appropriate Care to People With Intellectual and Developmental Disabilities 48
nursing
    definition of 1
    education 61–62
    essential documents xi–xii
    how 16–17, 41–43
    key influences 40–41
    standards of professional practice 8
    when 15–16
    where 29–39
    who 50–53
    why 41–43
    work environments 31–36
    workforce 59–61
Nursing Care for Individuals with Developmental Disabilities: An Integrated Approach 25
Nursing: Scope and Standards of Practice xi
nursingworld.org xii

O

ongoing assessment data 87
organizational resources 105
outcomes identification 9, 76–77

P

palliative care 45, 91
parent caregivers 67–68
parenting 67
patient handling and mobility 32–34
Pediatric Nursing: Scope and Standards of Practice xii
peer review 104
personal and professional development 47
person-centered care 76, 81
PhD (Doctor of Philosophy) degree 51
physical/behavioral skills 54
planning 9, 77–80
policymaking 97
popular media 108
population focus 65–67
population trends 60
positions
    academic consultation 52
    administrative 52
poster presentations 101
practice environment 36, 102, 106
practice portfolios 56
prescriptive authority 82
Principles for Nursing Documentation for Registered Nurses and Professional Nursing xiii
Principles of Environmental Health for Nursing Practice xiii
professional development 47, 62
professional nursing practice standards 71
professional practice evaluation 10, 103–104
Professional Role Competence: ANA Position Statement xiii
Psychiatric-Mental Health Nursing: Scope and Standards of Practice xii
public health 61
Public Health Nursing: Scope and Standards of Practice xii

Q

quality improvement projects 102
quality of practice 10, 54, 102–103

R

registered nurse 6–7, 50–53
    independent practice 41–42
rehabilitation 64
Rehabilitation Act of 1973 13, 49
rehabilitative technologies (RT) 64–65
relationship, nurse and individual with IDD 19, 45, 47, 88
research 26–28, 101
resource utilization 10, 104–106
responsibility 46–47
rights, protection of 49
risk factors 35, 107
risk-reducing behaviors 85
role models 37
RT (rehabilitative technologies) 64–65

S

safe patient handling and mobility (SPHM) 32–34
safe spaces 48
safety, culture of 32
Sawin, K. J. 28
SBAR (situation, background, assessment, and recommendation) 16
scholarly inquiry 48
school nurses 6–7
    IEPs and ITPs 15
    settings 30
School Nurses Working with Handicapped Children 25
School Nursing: Scope and Standards of Practice xii
science of IDD nursing
    evidence-based practice 28–29
    knowledge 22–26
    research 26–28
SDM. *See* informed shared decision-making (ISDM)
SDPB (Society for Developmental and Behavioral Pediatrics) 59
self-advocacy 46, 58
self-assessment 55
self-care 37, 83, 85, 89. *See also* care
self-determination 19, 46, 50, 89–90

self-evaluation 103
self-regulation 42
settings 15–16, 29–31
    deinstitutionalization movement 60
    different from other specialities 3
    school 30
    universities 30
sexuality 45, 90
shortages of healthcare workers 52–53, 60
situation, background, assessment, and recommendation (SBAR) 16
sleep health 34–35
smartphones 65
social justice 49–50, 91
Social Policy Statement: The Essence of the Profession 17
Society for Developmental and Behavioral Pediatrics (SDBP), Advanced Practice Clinician (APC) Section 59
Society of Adolescent Medicine 7
Society of Pediatric Nursing (SPN) 7
specialty practice 5–7
SPHM (safe patient handling and mobility) 32–34
SPN (Society of Pediatric Nursing) 7
staffing
    optimal 36
    shortages 52–53
Standards for the Clinical Advanced Practice Registered Nurse in Developmental Disabilities/Handicapping Conditions 25
Standards of Developmental Disabilities Nursing Practice 25
Standards of Nursing Practice in Mental Retardation/Developmental Disabilities 25
standards of practice 8–9, 48
standards of practice for IDD nurses 72–87
    assessment 72–74
    coordination of care 83–84
    diagnosis 74–76
    evaluation 86–87
    health teaching and health promotion 85–86
    implementation 80–83
    outcomes identification 76–77
    planning 77–80
standards of professional nursing practice 71
standards of professional performance for IDD nurses 9–10, 88–108
    collaboration 95–97
    communication 94–95
    culturally congruent practice 92–94
    education 99–100
    environmental health 106–108
    ethics 88–91
    evidence-based practice and research 100–101
    leadership 97–99
    professional practice evaluation 103–104
    quality of practice 102–103
    resource utilization 104–106
Statement on the Scope and Standards for the Nurse Who Specializes in Developmental Disabilities and/or Mental Retardation 25
statistics on IDD nurses 50–51
surrogate for healthcare decisions 46, 89. *See also* family
sustainable nursing workforce 59–61
synthesizing data and knowledge 73, 86

T

TeamSTEPPS 16
teamwork 40, 49, 96
technology 62–64, 105
    assistive 20, 63–64
    millennials and 65–66
    rehabilitative 64–65
    safe patient handling 33
telehealth services 58
terminology, offensive 22, 24

The Future of Disability in America, IOM Report 41

U
UAPs/UAFs (University-Affiliated Programs and Facilities) 23
UCEED (University Centers of Excellence in Developmental Disabilities Education, Research and Service) 51
underserved populations 53
University-Affiliated Programs and Facilities (UAPs or UAFs) 23
University Centers of Excellence in Developmental Disabilities Education, Research and Service (UCEDD) 51

V
violence 35–36, 48

W
Watson's framework 21
wheelchairs 33
WHO (World Health Organization) 72
work environments
    fatigue 34–35
    healthy 31–36, 47–48, 89
    staffing 36
    supports for 37–39
    violence and incivility 35–36, 48
workforce
    shortages 52
    sustainable nursing 59–61
World Health Organization (WHO) 72